WHAT PEOPLE ARE SAYING ABOUT

RECLAIMING YOURSELF FROM BINGE EATING

Leora Fulvio takes the mystery out of binge eating in her wonderful new book. *Reclaiming Yourself from Binge Eating* is readable, engaging and eye opening. Ms. Fulvio obviously cares about people who binge eat and knows how to help them stop, heal and reclaim personhood through health and freedom. I highly recommend this book.

Joanna Poppink, MFT, author of *Healing Your Hungry Heart: Recovering from Your Eating Disorder*

This book is a gift to people with Binge Eating Disorder and other forms of disordered eating. Leora Fulvio provides step-by-step practical, compassionate advice that by its nature will help the reader slow down, gain self-understanding and ultimately the self-acceptance necessary to make positive change. I will recommend this book enthusiastically to patients and friends alike.

Avril Swan, MD

Ms. Fulvio's voice is clear and comprehensive enough to replace the voice of the eating disorder. There are nuggets of wisdom in every paragraph.

Sheira Kahn, MFT, co-author of *The Erasing ED Treatment Manual*

D1111627

Reclaiming Yourself from Binge Eating

A Step-by-Step Guide to Healing

Reclaiming Yourself from Binge Eating

A Step-by-Step Guide to Healing

Leora Fulvio

AYNI BOOKS

Winchester, UK
Washington, USA

First published by Ayni Books, 2014
Ayni Books is an imprint of John Hunt Publishing Ltd., Laurel House, Station Approach,
Alresford, Hants, SO24 9JH, UK
office1@jhpbooks.net
www.johnhuntpublishing.com
www.ayni-books.com

For distributor details and how to order please visit the 'Ordering' section on our website.

ISBN: 978 1 78099 680 6

A CIP catalogue record for this book is available from the British Library.

Design: Lee Nash

Printed and bound by CPI Group (UK) Ltd, Croydon, CR0 4YY

We operate a distinctive and ethical publishing philosophy in all
areas of our business, from our global network of authors to
production and worldwide distribution.

CONTENTS

Medical Disclaimer

The information provided in this book is intended to educate you about Binge Eating Disorder and discusses different methods of healing. It is not a substitute for examination, diagnosis, and medical care provided by a licensed and qualified health professional. If you are suffering from an eating disorder, please do make an appointment to talk to your health care provider as well as a licensed Therapist or Psychologist.

Acknowledgements

Thank you to all my previous teachers, colleagues and supervisors, Victoria Green, Susie Finch, Nicole Laby, Linda McCabe, Ada Karlstrand and so many others whom I spent time in the trenches with. Thank you for your support, your patience and your wisdom. Thank you to all of my various yoga and meditation teachers throughout time. Thank you to my Mom and my Step-Mom, my two blessings. I miss you both every day. Thank you to my Dad and my brother who motivate me.

Thank you to every single patient. Each one of you have been my teachers. I appreciate your openness, honesty, your courage and willingness to be vulnerable. I love and value all of you.

Most of all, thank you to my husband, who has encouraged and supported me throughout this process and to my son and my son on the way; without them I'd never know that this level of love existed.

Part One

All About Binge Eating

Introduction

It started with the bread. It *always* started with the bread.

It was a Wednesday evening after work. Dusk was falling and the city streets were twinkling with that pre-holiday excitement. People were in and out of bars and restaurants, enjoying happy hour, enjoying each other and enjoying their lives.

But not me.

I blended in as I dragged myself home from work just trying to make it through the home stretch to my apartment. The smells from the corner bakery wafted up into my nose triggering intense grumblings from my stomach.

"Shut up, you," I grumbled back. "You're too big and fat to complain, get over yourself."

I had worked so hard all day. I just had to get past the bakery without stopping. Other than some wilted lettuce, a six-pack of Diet Coke and about 5 cups of coffee, I hadn't eaten anything at all. I held my breath as I walked past the bakery. I was on an all lettuce and tofu diet for the next 30 days. Bread was out. Cupcakes were out. Even fruit was out. But as I approached the bakery, I saw that they were taking the baguettes out of the oven. I looked away. Stupid bread, with its hard crust on the outside and soft, white, warm evil on the inside. I held my breath and walked right past the bakery.

Back at my apartment, I was greeted by a refrigerator that was mostly empty – I usually kept it that way. But I had gone shopping so there were several pouches of firm tofu and a head of lettuce. There was also half a bottle of chardonnay. The tofu seemed unappetizing, and I was absolutely bored of lettuce.

"Wine has no carbs," I thought. "Maybe I'll just have one glass to help me relax and perhaps sleep so that I don't have to think about food."

I poured myself a glass and settled in front of the television to watch some sitcoms and shake off the day. As I gulped the wine, my stomach grumbled. "Shut up, you," I said. I was starving. I sucked down the rest of the bottle and waited for sleep to set in. But drunkenness beat sleep and I stumbled aimlessly down to the corner store. I thought that I'd buy a pack of sleeping pills so that I could just pass out and defeat hunger.

Hunger was loud and strong – very, very loud. But I knew that if I could beat it tonight, tomorrow would be easier and eventually I would be in control. That was the game that I played with myself, or against myself. My hunger would fight with my self-control and discipline. The problem was, there were no winners in that game. If my self-control won, there I was – starving as my body ate itself. If my hunger won, I'd find myself stuffed in a corner, surrounded by food as I tried to eat my way out. It didn't really matter who won or who lost. I was losing the battle between a healthy mind and body, and a horrible eating disorder – sick body and sick mind.

How many women and men are fighting this battle constantly? We think it's a battle of wills, our self-control, our best disciplined self vs. our wild out of control glutton self. But that's not the battle we fight. Those of us who have been living with disordered eating are holding a place for healthy thoughts, bodies and self-esteems to duke it out with this pervasive sickness that seems to be a virus in this society. The "There is something very wrong with me" virus.

On that particular night, my eating disorder won again. It didn't matter if I chose to go to the store and binge or if I wound up falling asleep into a subtle coma of sleeping pills, wine and hunger; the eating disorder won.

If it hadn't, perhaps I would have broken out of this cycle, this coma, and chosen health. Perhaps I would have put the wine down, prepared a healthy and satisfying meal and gotten over it. But that's not what happened. That night, I walked down to the store, bought a pack of over-the-counter sleeping pills which I took while I was still in the store; I bought another bottle of wine and gave in and grabbed one of those baguettes. I told myself that I'd only have one small piece of the bread. But I began eating it in the store as I walked through and ate much more than my allotment of one small piece. That's it. My night was already ruined. So I went ahead and grabbed a box of pasta, some sauce, brie, and a packet of Oreos. At home, behind closed doors, I drank another glass of wine as I prepared a giant pot of spaghetti. After I finished off a whole box of spaghetti and the warm, crusty bread and the pack of Oreos, I fell into an uncomfortable but deep sleep. I woke up in the morning hungover and hating myself, vowing that today would be different. And the cycle continued. Not every night ended with me bingeing and passing out. There were some nights when I'd chase my meals with some ex-lax and wait for the food to pass, and many nights when I didn't eat a thing and passed out hungrily, waking up the next morning feeling empty and proud of myself. That could go on for days. But eventually I would get hungry. This cycle lasted for years longer than I wish it had. Sometimes I mourn for the years I lost to food and food games and wars against my body.

My story begins before my eating disorder ever began.

I was four years old when I attended my first Weight Watchers® meeting with my mom. We weren't there for me; we were there for her. I don't remember what happened at the meeting, I was too fixated on the TAB® Cola machines. I lay on the floor in the back of the meeting room and stared up at the machine, longing and fantasizing. My mom didn't let me have soda and the bounty above was hypnotic. There was every flavor of TAB® imaginable. Orange Tab®, Lemon Lime Tab®, Root Beer Tab®, even Cherry Tab®. Before the meeting started, my mom would purchase one to sip throughout the meeting, usually root beer. It was the only time she let herself drink soda. My mother was thin. Not stick thin, but she was a small woman. She had a tiny waist and small bones, but she had strong, solid thighs and amazing childbearing hips, which, fortunately for my son, I inherited. She dieted and dieted and dieted. She got bonier and thinner all over her body except for in her hips and thighs, and disparaged herself for it. This was not what she, an aspiring ballerina, desired for herself.

As I began to develop a body, my mother noticed that I too had thighs like her own – strong, short, and thick. These were good for the things I liked to do, like run, swim, do gymnastics and generally be sporty. But my mother, because of her own body hatred, felt compelled to make them stop before they started. She was appalled when we went shopping at Wanamaker's to find that, at 11 years old, she had to buy me a junior size seven pants. "That's a woman's size! Not a little girl's size!"

I attended my first Weight Watchers® meeting as a participant at the age of 11. I was 95 pounds and my mother was determined to get me to 85. It worked. That's how I learned about calories, restricting and bingeing. By the time I was 13, I was back at Weight Watchers®. But this time I was a little older, had a little more independence and was not going to fall prey to my mother's dry tuna, cottage cheese and cantaloupe regime. I realized that if I went the whole day without eating, I would have enough "exchanges" left by the end of the day for a Three Musketeers and a Snickers. Breakfast and lunch were skipped, and I would tell my mom that I was having dinner at a friend's or out at the diner. Instead, I'd binge on candy bars. And it worked. I seemed to lose weight that way. At school, I gravitated toward the skinny fashionable mean girls and wanted to do whatever I could to fit in with them. I wanted to be thin. I wanted to wear the best jeans. I wanted acceptance and love. I certainly wasn't giving it to myself.

I managed my weight by adopting a vegetarian diet, which eventually became a vegan diet. Yet, it wasn't enough for me to control myself; and so at fourteen years old, I began smoking cigarettes to decrease my appetite and control my eating. This was the late 1980s. There was no misinformation about smoking. I knew it was deadly. But it didn't matter. Being thin was all that mattered. This began a binge-restrict cycle that lasted for years.

In high school, I wouldn't eat anything all day long. Then I'd get home and binge on chips, brownies, milkshakes, French fries, and candy. Often I'd buy food out and about, and find a deserted place in my neighborhood where I could sit alone and eat. Sometimes I would take laxatives, other times I'd exercise compulsively and yet other times after eating furiously, I would just go home, climb into bed and pass out without any compensation at all and vow to start a diet the next day. This behavior continued well into college, and even into my 20s. Eventually, food was replaced with wine. No food all day, then in the evenings, to prevent bingeing, I just drank wine and snacked on chips and salsa. Obsession with food, exercise, and the constant pursuit of thinness took over my life. I wasn't interested in much else and I based my happiness on how thin I was and what kind of clothes I could fit into. It was quite a miserable existence. Sure I was doing other things, I had a life outside of my eating issues, I had hobbies, I dated and even had relationships – albeit not successful or even functional ones. I had my education and my work and my friends, but I was pretty good at keeping my issues to myself. I didn't discuss food or bingeing with anyone. And even though I pretended to be engaged in life, my brain was just wrapped around food and how to get thin. I had a secret life inside my head. I'd be out with friends and outwardly we'd be discussing something deeply important but in my head, I'd be plotting and calculating: "1/2 bagel with inside scooped out – 125 calories, light cream cheese – 50 calories, milk in my coffee – 25 calories..." I spent my time smoking cigarettes, concentrating on not eating, running on a treadmill, and drunk. And all those hours running, all those meals rejected, all of those laxatives, cigarettes, bottles of wine, and still – I had my mother's thighs.

The strong, thick thighs I was predestined to have.

I'm not tall. I'm barely 5'2". I can't change my height. I know that. But trying to would have been as insane as trying to change the shape of my body. No matter how thin I got, my body would retain the same shape. Yet, somehow, I thought that if I were just disciplined enough, I could have the body of Elle Macpherson. It was crazy-making.

Why did I waste all that time? Aren't there so many other things I could have been thinking about or doing? Aren't there so many relationships I could have been cultivating? Couldn't I have been on a career trajectory?

Obsessing about food and my body kept me from living my life. But it was safe in a strange way. I always believed that my life would start when I lost the weight that I wanted to lose. The truth is though, that my life had started a long time ago and I was actively choosing not to be a part of it. I was afraid and I was shutting down with food, alcohol, cigarettes and exercise.

My recovery came in four parts.

First, I had to relearn how to eat regular meals. Eventually, I even began to eat an omnivore diet. That might not be the right thing for everyone, but I felt better physically. I began to eat three meals each day. I learned to eat when I was hungry and stop when I was satisfied. No foods were off limits; however, I had to learn how to use boundaries with food to allow myself what I wanted without going overboard and hurting myself with it. Although I was not even close to being perfect, I had to learn to accept that and remember that I always had the next meal to try again. I practiced giving my body what it needed and tried to honor it most of the time with healthy whole foods.

Second, I learned how to distinguish real hunger from boredom, sadness, loneliness and anxiety. Then, I had to learn how to sit with these feelings without judgment and to allow myself to feel what I needed to feel. Understanding that feelings, all of them, were okay was what really helped me to cope with them without food and without avoiding.

Third, I began to use mindfulness and meditation to learn how to stop myself and interrupt the compulsive behavior. I began by just watching. I took a step back and didn't get in my own way. I watched myself make choices to do things that were either good for me or bad for me. As I learned how to take a step back and just be aware of what I was doing, I was in a better position to actually make choices about my behavior and not allow the compulsion to make them for me.

Fourth, I had to learn how to accept my body the way it is, thighs and all. I began to see that I was more than a body. I was a mind, a spirit, a soul, a being, and I had a lot to offer – my value wasn't tied up in the size of my jeans. After having my son, I felt even more in awe of my body. It didn't seem like a showpiece anymore. It was a real, utilitarian piece of machinery. It not only created and grew a whole human being, it continued to make food to keep him alive and help him thrive for a very long time. In fact, I began to wonder why women's bodies were objectified when they are such workhorses. I mused that men's nipples were vestigial – why weren't they all over magazines trying to sell items?

As I learned to like myself, my life got much, much better. My mother had been so concerned with what other people thought of her that everything she did was for the benefit of others to make them like her. She thought she could control what others thought of her by controlling her body. She thought that if she had a certain type of body people would think of her in a certain way. When she saw that I had a similar body to her, she thought that she was helping me by starting me on a diet so early. She thought that if I didn't get her thighs, I wouldn't have to go through what she went through; I wouldn't have to worry about whether or not people liked me if I was thin or beautiful. The problem, though, was that I never got time to think about whether or not I liked me. I didn't get to know myself. As I let go of my eating issues and began to focus on me, I became so much more solid. There were little things that I did that helped me to have boundaries and to have parameters so that my life felt in control. I made sure that I made my bed every morning. I ate breakfast, lunch and dinner every single day. I flossed my teeth at night and I went to bed before midnight. As long as I kept those boundaries, I had something to fall back on in order to rein it in when I felt out of control with food. These little things helped me to feel solid and grounded. They gave me the containment to pursue other interests. Within this containment I was able to recover from my eating disorder, go to graduate school for psychology and counsel women at an intensive outpatient treatment center for eating disorders recovery. I was able to travel, write, read, form and maintain fulfilling friendships and find an amazing person to share my life with. Life opened up for me once I let go of the eating disorder and let myself into my life.

Chapter One

Using This Book

This is not a diet book, nor is this a weight loss book, though weight loss may be an incidental part of the healing process as you let go of binge eating. This is a mind, body and spirit book, that utilizes mindfulness and self-acceptance in order to help you heal on every level.

The book has an action plan, specific external steps that you should take to help yourself stop binge eating, and it also has more internal steps to help you increase your awareness and understand why you binge eat. Finally, it has exercises and meditations that will completely change the way you think and behave around food.

In addition to this book, make sure to have a notebook or journal on hand. During the course of the book, when it is advisable to write through the steps, you will see the phrase *Journal Opportunity*. If you would prefer to go through the book and go back to do your steps after you've read it, you can do that too. You can also find a journal with all the writing prompts at www.reclaimingyourselffrombingeeating.com. There is no prescribed formula. Just find what works for you. You might find that just one or two steps click for you and help you to completely give up binge eating, and you might find that different chapters resonate for you at different times in your life. You can return to things at certain times in your life when they have more relevance and learn something different from them then.

Throughout the book, you will also see the phrase *Meditation Time*. At this time, you can read the meditation, then close your eyes and focus on the specific meditation that is relevant to the chapter. Each of these meditations is also available for download at the website if you would prefer to be guided through the meditations.

Besides a journal, I also recommend having a support person on hand while you are working through this book. You can use this book with a therapist, a friend, a 12-step sponsor, you can create a Reclaiming Yourself from Binge Eating group, or you can just use it by yourself. It's encouraged to have at least one support person on hand so that you don't have to do certain exercises alone. You might feel that some of the chapters or the exercises don't resonate with you or are not relevant to your situation. That's okay. You don't have to do every step. Some might just feel that they are not for you. Just do what makes you comfortable and what your *wise mind* (more on that in Chapter Eight) tells you is right for you. This is about finding yourself and learning to meet your needs without food. You might find that you come back to certain exercises later and notice that they resonate with you more than they did when you first looked at them.

I do not recommend reading this book all in one sitting. You could do a step every few days, once a week, once a month or even more. Take time to metabolize it, to be with it, to think about it, to discuss it with your support people, or just spend time thinking or journaling about what's coming up for you. There is no urgency when it comes to recovery. It's about slowly coming back to yourself, getting to know you in a deep meaningful way.

The book is divided into two sections. The first section is about understanding Binge Eating Disorder. The next section is a step-by-step guide on exactly how to stop binge eating. The first steps are action steps. They give you very specific actions to change your behaviors. The next steps are internal steps. They are meant to help you think about your relationship to food, your body, the people around you and how they all relate to binge eating issues. At the end, there are appendixes with all your tools. These are your worksheets, your meditations and some quick references for you.

Letting go of Binge Eating Disorder is usually not a quick fix. It is a rich process of increasing awareness at the same time as you change behaviors, a glorious exercise in patience and self-acceptance. The great news is that you begin to have insight into who you are and why you do what you do, and gain new and different behaviors that help you to feel better and like yourself more. These changes are lifelong because they come from within.

Healing from Binge Eating Disorder is like breaking up with someone who you have been in a dysfunctional relationship with. In some ways, food has been your best friend or your lover. It has always been there for you, has always comforted you, and unlike people, food consistently made you feel better when you were down. But then comes the letdown. The after-binge feeling, when you feel worse than you did before you binged. Just like leaving that dysfunctional relationship, you might experience sadness or grief after letting go of the disorder. However, the freedom that you experience when you are out of this relationship with food will give you strength, health, and a more fulfilling life. Imagine yourself being who you want to be, in the body you want to be in, feeling the way you want to feel, looking forward to things other than eating, enjoying other parts of life, having the confidence that you want to have. It can all be yours. Of course, this doesn't come magically by reading a book, going to a seminar, listening to a recording, or taking a pill. You have habits and coping mechanisms that have been ingrained into your psyche since early childhood. These coping mechanisms are behaviors that used to work beautifully, but no longer serve you.

For instance, a young patient of mine, Liz, remembers that as a child her mother and father would fight incessantly. In order to escape their wrath, she would sit in her room and eat cookies and listen to music to drown out the noise and distract herself. She became so anxious when they fought, fearing that her parents would divorce and she'd be without one of them. The cookies made her feel better. She described it as completely calming the tension inside of her. However, now, as a 25-year-old woman, whenever there is any conflict around her, she instantly turns to food. So, at work, when her boss says something that she doesn't like, she feels unable to speak up for herself and runs to the cafe downstairs for a latté and a pastry. If her boyfriend does something like spend the night with his friends instead of her, rather than discuss it with him, she binges on cookies. This reaction was for a long time not conscious. However, through awareness, mindfulness exercises, and tracking, she was able to understand what was causing these binges.

"But I had a great day!" she once told me. "I have no idea why I ate a whole box of cookies by myself, I just wanted them. Everything was fine before that." We went through the day in a very detailed way. She did mention offhandedly that she put her headphones on at one point because her officemate was loudly arguing with her boyfriend on the phone.

"How did that make you feel?" I asked her.

"It didn't make me feel anything," she said, "but I didn't want to hear that. I just put my headphones on and drowned out the noise of the arguing."

"Like the way you used to sit in your room with the music turned up to drown out the sound of your parents fighting?"

"It's completely different," she told me. "I don't care one bit if Charlotte is fighting with her boyfriend. I don't even like Charlotte, she's very annoying."

"So, when you hear Charlotte fighting with her boyfriend, you feel…"

"Annoyed."

"Anything else?"

"Angry."

"What else?"

"I just don't want to hear it."

"You just don't want to hear it. But Charlotte's relationship with her boyfriend has nothing to do with you."

"It's distracting. I had to hear enough of that with my mom and dad. I don't want to hear it in my workplace."

"Ah, so you cope with it in the same way as you did when you were a little girl."

"I guess I do."

Liz had found a way to deal with the fear of her parents divorcing as a child by listening to music, bingeing and tuning out. As an adult, she found that she repeated the same behavior.

Liz began to carefully track her binges and identify what happened on the days that she would binge. Using mindfulness, she began to understand when she was being triggered. She also understood that this was old information and no longer useful to her. She began to learn how to have healthy confrontations and boundaries, which enriched her relationships and helped her binges to subside completely. She didn't give up cookies; however, she found that she was able to eat one or two rather than 30–40 in a sitting.

Usually, there is more than one simple reason for people to binge. They are complicated and compounded by several different issues often rooted in family, self-esteem, body image, the fear or inability to sit with uncomfortable feelings, physical issues, biological, chemical and genetic reasons. It takes work to conquer all of these, but it is completely possible. I know that people who do the work are handsomely rewarded with a feeling of calmness and peace around food, and an overall feeling of emotional well-being.

Chapter Two

What is Mindfulness and How Will It Help Me Heal?

Buddhist teachings consider mindfulness a path toward enlightenment. This means *a daily conscious awareness of your thoughts, feelings, physical sensations, bodily functions, movements, actions, reactions, beliefs, fears, anxieties and drives.*

When you are mindful, you are present and aware. You are aware of your feelings and your bodily sensations, your emotional and your physical needs. When you are mindless, you are multitasking, you are drinking coffee and eating a bagel while driving the kids to school, you are fiddling with your iPhone, watching television, and eating lunch all at once. You are browsing the Internet while talking to your mom or checking your e-mail while nursing your baby. While we live in a society where multitasking is rewarded and often necessary, it seems that we can lose sight of who we are and what we are doing when there is just too much happening. When you are mindless, you are not present, and you don't notice what you need and why you are doing what you are doing. Your current task takes on momentum and then you follow the 'doing' rather than making active choices about what you need. When you do not integrate any mindfulness at all into your tasks, you might find that you move through your day almost automatically, driving to and from work and completing your daily tasks without noticing how you got there. All of a sudden, you're at the office; all of a sudden, you've eaten lunch; all of a sudden, it's 10pm; you've come home from work, eaten, watched three hours of television and it's time for bed. Your life passes without you being an active participant in it. Without mindfulness, bingeing chooses you rather than you choosing it. Because you are not actively engaged in your choices, you barely have time to make the decision not to binge. You barely have a moment to notice what you are feeling.

Mindfulness helps to decrease binge eating by helping you to fully experience all of your emotions, the joyful ones and the hard ones. By letting yourself feel your feelings, even the really difficult ones, you increase your capacity for sitting with painful and even distressing moods, thoughts and sensations. When you are more able to sit with these feelings, you don't feel driven to do something about it. There is nothing to be done with feelings other than feel them.

Creating a mindfulness practice will give you the tools to pause, notice what you are feeling, notice what you want to do in reaction to that feeling, and allow you just a little bit of space to make that choice willingly. Being mindful gives you the opportunity to be more engaged in your life day-to-day, minute-by-minute. You don't have to be hyperaware of what you are doing every second for the rest of your life. However, by increasing your awareness, just a little bit each day, you become an active participant in your life. You then can create some more choice as to whether or not you want to binge. You can begin to understand why you are bingeing; you can choose alternatives to bingeing.

It's so easy to begin a mindfulness practice. Start slowly by setting an alarm on your phone to go off a few times a day. Each time the alarm goes off, stop whatever you are doing and take two deep breaths. Then ask yourself, "What am I feeling?" Simply name that feeling without any judgments attached to it, without labeling the feeling as good or bad. You might notice that you are feeling anxious. You don't have to do anything to change the anxiety. Just quietly say to yourself, "Anxious," and notice the feeling. That is a very basic way to begin creating mindfulness in your life. You might then go on to ask yourself, "Does this feeling put me at risk for a binge?" You have just increased your chance of being able to prevent a binge behavior. You might then sit and take a few moments (1–5 minutes) to do some very light meditation. You can close your eyes, or keep them open and unfocused, put your hand over your heart and tune in to your heartbeat, then just notice your breath. This simple act will bring you into the present moment. It connects you with yourself. Increasing mindfulness increases awareness; when you are aware of your actions, it decreases the chance that you will do something that will hurt you. This is because we often do things to make feelings go away. For instance, you might be at work and on a tight deadline which you have a great deal of stress about. You might then run to the kitchen and chow down on some cookies and coffee before you get started. If you were able to stop, acknowledge that you are stressed, take a few deliberate breaths into your belly and allow yourself to slow down, you might find that you don't need to go into the kitchen at all. In fact, you might be able to calm yourself down just by taking space to breathe. When you feel stress, your nervous system goes into overdrive and you begin shallow breathing – or chest breathing. You can switch off the fight-or-flight response by voluntarily moving from chest breathing to belly breathing. When you do this, you switch off the fight/flight response by changing your breathing from fast and shallow chest breathing to slow, steady diaphragmatic breathing. This sends a signal to your brain that the threat is over and the parasympathetic part of the Autonomic Nervous system starts to reverse the biochemical and physiological changes brought about by the fight/flight response. Diaphragmatic breathing works quickly and effectively. In fact, by taking belly breaths, you can slow down your heart rate, increase your blood flow, and relax your mind and body in about 60 seconds. Try it now.

Meditation Time
Start by lying in a relaxed position. Place one hand on your belly and one hand on your chest. The goal here is to send

your breath into your belly, not into your chest, so you should find that your belly expands but your chest remains relatively still. You don't have to take deep uncomfortable breaths, just let yourself find the natural flow of your breathing. Allow your breathing to be comfortable and to settle into its own rhythm. Let yourself continue to just watch your breath as you breathe into your belly for a minute. You can stay there longer, but after a minute the relaxation response should kick in. Using breath to create tranquility is the simplest and most natural way to relax. Our breath is a gift to us, an internal mechanism that is part of our design for creating peace. If you can just sit and breathe, you've found meditation. When you create time to do this every day, you will change your life by giving yourself a tool inside of you to help you manage your emotions.

The exercises in this book are set up to help you look closely at why you might be making certain choices. They are designed to help you think about why you made the choices that you did in the past, and why you continue to make certain choices. They will help you to take control over your behaviors. Once you have consciousness, once you know why you are willingly doing something, you then have awareness and choice and you are no longer controlled by the binge.

Chapter Three

Understanding Binge Eating Disorder

Binge Eating Disorder is the most common eating disorder in both the United States and the United Kingdom. It affects 3.5% of females and 2% of men.[1] The diet and weight loss industry might have you believe that curing binge eating disorder is a matter of willpower, and that certain diets can cure binge eating. However, binge eating is not something that is receptive to dieting. In fact, diets are one of the huge triggers of binge eating. Yet, people continue to get stuck in the cycle of binge eating, dieting, then binge eating again. The purpose of this book is to address and heal the underlying issues that lead to Binge Eating Disorder in order to empower people to release themselves from the continual trap of bingeing and dieting. Binge Eating Disorder is distinguished by the following:

Recurrent episodes of binge eating, which are characterized by the following:

You eat a very large amount of food when you are not physically hungry.

You eat more than your body needs, cautiously, secretly and quickly.

You feel as though you cannot control what and how much you are eating, and that you have no power to stop.

You eat lots of food rapidly and furiously.

You eat until you feel uncomfortably full and sometimes even ill.

You eat alone or hide with your food.

You feel disgusted with yourself, depressed, or very guilty after eating.

You act out in this behavior at least twice per week for at least three months.

However, you still can have issues with binge eating without meeting these exact criteria. Though guilt and shame can be indicative of a binge-eating episode, many women feel guilty, ashamed or angry with themselves after eating a normal amount of food or eating 'forbidden' foods. I worked with one patient who was so afraid of carbohydrates that she believed eating one bagel was a binge and punished herself accordingly by either restricting, excessive exercise, purging, or simply hate-filled self-talk. When it comes to disordered eating, it's difficult to know what is real and what isn't. Is it really a binge? Or is it normal and okay to eat a small bag of chips with your sandwich at lunchtime? Disordered eaters usually start off as dieters. On these diets they learn about certain foods that are okay to eat and others that are restricted. Some restrict carbohydrates, some restrict fat, and some set parameters for not going above a certain amount of calories. Usually, a chronic dieter will happen to eat a small amount of the food that he or she deems off limits, or go above their calorie limit. This might turn into a binge, or it might turn into a guilt festival, where the dieter feels bad about him or herself for eating the food that she or he had previously banished. It then becomes a moral issue. "I ate an avocado, and therefore I am a bad person." The dieter feels as though their inability to control themselves is what makes them bad.

What is a Binge?

A binge is eating more food than you're hungry for *and not being able to stop*. When it happens, you might feel as though you have no idea how you got there. Many people binge in a daze or a trance or feel unconscious, as if in some kind of dream state. Some just 'wake up' in the middle of a binge.

While most people tend to binge on carbohydrate-laden foods such as cereal, breads, ice cream, pizza, pastries, cookies, chocolate, donuts, pasta, and other heavy foods, that is not always the case. I've seen many people suffering with Binge Eating Disorder who tend to binge on meat or beans and rice, tofu, fruit and vegetables and other healthy foods. Binge Eating Disorder is not about the food, it's about how much food you are eating at one time and the feeling associated with the act of eating. If you are eating when you are not hungry, you are eating to achieve a different feeling.

A huge part of healing from Binge Eating Disorder is learning how to distinguish real bodily hunger from fake hunger – understanding when you are hungry for fuel or when you are using food to deal with anxiety, stress, anger, sadness, loneliness, emptiness or something else.

Quiz: How Do I Know if I am a Binge Eater?

1. Do you eat in secret?
2. Do you restrict certain foods sometimes but binge on them at other times?
3. Do you go off and on diets repeatedly?
4. Do you obsessively read health and fitness magazines and diet books?
5. Do you drink a lot of coffee or diet soda to keep you from eating?
6. Do you eat a certain way in front of people and completely differently when you're alone?
7. Do you steal, hide or hoard food?
8. Do you eat when you are not hungry?
9. Do you eat until you are uncomfortably full?
10. Do you feel guilt and shame after you eat something you think you shouldn't?
11. Do you ever try to compensate for what you've eaten by

exercising excessively, taking laxatives, throwing up, or restricting food the next day?

12. Do you often say things like, "This is the last time I'm going to eat this way, I'm starting my diet tomorrow."

13. Do you avoid certain situations because of food?

14. Do you avoid certain situations because you feel uncomfortable in your body?

15. Do you feel as though you can't stop when you start eating certain foods?

16. Do you think about food much of the time?

17. Do you eat when you are sad, lonely, anxious, tired, scared or bored?

18. Do you ever feel unsatisfied after a meal, even if you know that you are no longer hungry, and still try to find some kind of taste or meal that will satisfy you?

19. Do you justify your use of food as a reward or as medicine, such as, "Well, I'm sad today, it's okay for me to eat these cupcakes."

20. Do you justify your use of food because it's a special occasion, "My best friend who I never see is in town! It's necessary to eat this food at this restaurant!"

21. Do you often eat large amounts of food in inappropriate places such as in bed or in the car?

22. Do you find yourself scavenging for food? Searching for something to satisfy a certain urge and continuing to eat until you've found it?

If you said yes to one or more of these questions, chances are you probably engage in binge eating. If you said yes to 3 or more of these questions, it's likely that you are suffering from Binge Eating Disorder.

Disordered Eater vs. Eating Disorder

"But I don't have an eating disorder! I just make poor choices, and sometimes I overeat."

Is it possible to have disordered eating and not have an eating disorder? What's the difference? Yes, it is definitely possible to have disordered eating but not a full-blown eating disorder.

Eating disorders tend to be pervasive. Having an eating disorder invades and permeates every fiber of your being and it attacks you on every level, physically, emotionally, socially, spiritually, and mentally. Your eating disorder becomes your obsession. You find that you are unable to do the things that you used to enjoy, like go to parties, or dinners, or home to your parents' house – anywhere that food will be involved or that you will be tempted to eat. You find that you're unable to go to places that you had in the past out of the fear that people will silently criticize you for the way your body looks or that you will just feel uncomfortable in your body and not want to be out in public. You tend to avoid people and things that you used to enjoy in order to spend more time alone with your eating disorder. It is your world. You might avoid seeing people that you haven't seen in a long time for fear that they will notice and judge your weight. You begin to think that everyone is noticing your weight and the way you look. You forget that people have things to think about that are not your weight because you are so obsessed with it that you cannot see past it, and so you begin to avoid people. Your eating disorder becomes the center of your world, and very few things are more important. Your free time is spent acting out the behaviors of your eating disorder. You might also find that you are doing extreme things with food like stealing it, hiding it, hoarding it, sneak eating, starving yourself, stuffing yourself, purging after eating... And that these behaviors become your new best friend, your evil lover who you hate and love at the same time and can't seem to get rid of.

Disordered eating is more like a neurotic, yet inconsistent obsession with food and/or exercise that comes and goes. These are your diet addicts. You know them, people who always seem to be trying out a new diet, always talking about "when they're going to lose the weight." These people have an unhealthy relationship with food and their bodies yet they haven't necessarily taken it to an extreme to the point that it's all encompassing. As children, we all know how to eat to make our bodies run efficiently. However, that changes. Although children inherently know how to listen to their bodies, when processed foods, high fructose corn syrup, diet sodas and other 'non-food food items' are introduced and coupled with parents either forcing their children to eat or not letting them eat – you then have a kid who grows up into someone who has no idea what his or her body needs.[2] So they turn to outside sources, such as diet plans, to tell them what they should be eating rather than turning inward, to that deep, intuitive place that they are born with that tells them what their body needs.

Disordered eating, unfortunately, plagues a great deal of this country. Much of it stems from the fact that our food isn't food – it's overprocessed and doesn't innately resonate with our bodily cues for what we need. Socially, because we're conditioned to think that we're not okay if we are not super thin and toned like a Hollywood starlet, we automatically believe that something is wrong with us and that we're doing the wrong thing. That then creates a schism in our eating habits. Rather than intuitive, healthy eating for life and vitality, we begin haphazard, disordered eating in hopes of being thin.

Chapter Four

Why Do I Binge Eat?

There are as many reasons for people to have Binge Eating Disorder as there are different personalities. And there is rarely just one reason that can be pointed to.

Physiological Influences

Through twin studies and by isolating the MC4R gene, it has been shown that there is a genetic link that might contribute to binge eating.[3] The MC4 receptors are involved in feeding and metabolic regulation. In 1998, it was found that mutations on the MC4R gene were associated with inherited obesity. One such study hypothesizes that the hypothalamus (the part of the brain that controls appetite) may not be sending correct messages about hunger and fullness.[4] In some studies, researchers found a genetic mutation that appears to cause food addiction.[5] It has been found that food addiction follows the same neural pathways that are active in drug addition.[6] There is also evidence that serotonin deficiencies, which cause depression, also contribute to binge eating.[7] It is also probable that continued bingeing and restricting can adversely affect brain chemistry and serotonin levels thus leading to depression.[8]

Psychological Influences

A strong correlation has been found between binge eating and depression.[9] According to the US Department of Health and Human Services, close to 50% of binge eaters are either currently suffering from depressive disorders or had previously. The evidence indicates that failing self-esteem, loneliness and body dissatisfaction or even body hatred are largely involved in Binge Eating Disorder. People with Binge Eating Disorder may also have trouble with impulse control as well as emotional regulation or managing and expressing their feelings.[10]

Social Influences

External influences, such as family and societal pressure to be thin, can also increase feelings of shame that binge eaters feel which can then fuel their emotional eating. The irony here is that the binge eater, when what she needs most is compassion and understanding, will self-soothe by binge eating and then berate herself for failing. This feedback loop is continuous.

Binge Eating Disorder can also be formed when parents use food to control their children. They give them certain types of food, usually a 'treat' like cookies to calm them when they are upset, to dismiss them when they are busy, to bribe them or reward them for good behavior. This forms a roadmap for those children to use food when they are sad, happy, rejected or bored. As adults, they begin to see food as something to calm them when they become upset, or something to go to when they are bored, or even something to turn to in times of celebration or happiness as a reward.

Children with parents who are hypercritical toward their bodies and try to control their food are at risk of developing Binge Eating Disorder. They feel unsafe eating in front of their parents, or eating anything that is not 'virtuous', so they will eat in secret, sometimes snatching restricted food from the refrigerator or even stealing food and eating it alone in private.

Coping Mechanism

Some people use food to fill chronic emptiness. Others eat out of boredom, to add some excitement into their worlds. Some people use food to stuff down feelings that are too uncomfortable to feel. And then there are all the reasons that people obsess on food. What are they avoiding? If they weren't thinking about food, what would they be thinking about? They use food or the constant goal of weight loss to focus on something other than their real lives. Their lives become about food, weight and their diets. Other things, thoughts and activities fall by the wayside, only to be usurped by the omnipresent obsession with losing weight.

Longing

Pain and misery is often caused by obsessing on something that you don't have. As you continue to focus on what you don't have, you begin to feel hopeless, sad, depressed and obsessed. Wanting something that you don't have is painful. Obsessing on something you don't have is devastating. This can be something as innocuous as being depressed because you don't have the kind of money you need to buy the kind of car that you want to drive or as deeply felt as not having a serious relationship or a life partner. Sometimes filling the void of something that you can't have with something that you can easily have, like a cupcake, can momentarily make you feel better. But then, it makes you feel worse. The pain of bingeing alone coupled with not having what you want or believe you should have can be isolating and overwhelming. Happiness is challenging when you are sitting alone focused on what you don't have. Of course it's necessary to have goals and to have something that you're striving for. Goals are imperative to your happiness and well-being. However, when goals become obsessions, it's impossible to be appreciative of the moment. How can you be happy where you are when you are obsessed with being somewhere or something else? Being comfortable does not mean being complacent. It's totally possible to be happy and have goals to move forward. At the same time, it's crucial for your overall happiness and well-being that you can have some gratitude and love for what you do have in the moment. As long as you obsess on what you don't have and forget about what you have, you will never find inner peace.

For instance, dwelling on a skinny body when your body is

curvy will only cause you to feel insignificant and insecure. Being able to embrace your body at the size that it is will not only make you happier, but it will enable you to take care of it lovingly. You take care of things and people that you love, not that you hate. When you hate your body, you treat it poorly. Bingeing, purging, starving and dieting are punishing behaviors that you inflict on your body for it not being what you think it should be. When you love your body, you care for it, you feed it healthy food without overfeeding it and you exercise it appropriately. Try to change your thinking by shifting your focus slightly when you are feeling 'in the want' to gratitude for what you currently have. You can still be striving for what you want without living in the anger of not having it.

Perceived Powerlessness

One of the things that we rarely remember in recovery is that we actually have a choice. Sometimes, when we have the urge to binge, it feels like we have no choice whatsoever. If we have the urge, we have to do it. But the truth is, you always have a choice. If you are feeling the urge to binge, you can decide not to. Just because you want it doesn't mean you have to have it. Mindfulness training teaches us to notice desire as a fleeting feeling, one that doesn't have to be satisfied. So, for instance, when you are having a craving for a binge food or the urge to binge, letting yourself notice that you are craving, letting yourself be with the urge without letting the urge satisfy itself is the way to increase your capacity for sitting with cravings. Just because you want to eat doesn't mean that you have to. You can allow want to be there, and allow yourself to feel uncomfortable with that feeling. Yes, it will be challenging to sit with the anxiety of wanting to but choosing not to binge. It can feel like an unscratchable itch, and the only way to relieve it is to binge. However, you can allow yourself some discomfort and some anxiety. The more often you allow yourself to sit with the discomfort of an urge without satisfying the urge, the stronger you become. This is how you begin to reclaim yourself from binge eating. You are in charge and you are in power, not the urge, not the binge. Anxiety and discomfort and desire and even feeling the intense need to binge are just feelings. Feelings cannot and will not kill you. You can sit with these. Sometimes it can feel like you are just jumping out of your skin. And in the past that is just what you have done: you ran to food to make that feeling go away. Acknowledging that it's difficult, but that it's okay for you to go through some difficulty, can help you move through and get to the other side.

I met Julie when I was working at a treatment facility for eating disorders. At the end of each of our sessions, just as our time was up, Julie would end by threatening that she was going to order a pizza and eat the whole thing by herself. When I first began working with her, I would go over our time and make suggestions for ways to keep herself safe from that pizza. Nothing ever worked; she'd go home, order the pizza and eat the whole pie. One night, when I was particularly tired and in no place to stay overtime, she threatened me again.

"Well, Julie," I said, "if you're going to eat the pizza, eat the pizza, I can't stop you. This is your choice."

"You're not going to try to stop me?" she asked incredulously.

"No," I told her. "There's nothing I can do. I'm not the one steering this ship. It's time I trust you to make your own choices."

The next day when I checked in on her, she told me that she hadn't binged the night before.

"How come not last night?" I asked her.

"Well," she said, "last night, for the first time, I realized that I actually had a choice. So I chose not to."

"How was that for you?" I asked her.

"It was really, really, really hard. But I did it. And I know I can do it again."

I set boundaries with her, which then gave her the example of how to set boundaries with herself. Although she did binge again, that was the real beginning of her recovery; her awareness had kicked in and she knew that she was the one in charge and that she could set boundaries, the pizza wasn't the boss of her.

Dwelling on the Past

Binge eaters can often forget that they only have forward to go. They spend a lot of time trying to undo a binge. Rather than focusing on their next meal, it's either, "Okay, I screwed up by bingeing, or eating the wrong food, I am going to spend the rest of the day eating as much of whatever I want..." Or, alternately, "Oh no, I binged, I can't eat anything except for water until Thursday..." instead of saying to themselves, "Okay. I had a rough morning with food. But it doesn't have to continue. I can relax and make my next meal a healthy one." The sense of not going forward keeps the binge and the bingeing behavior with them and the cycle continues.

Resistance

I started smoking cigarettes at 14 years old. I started trying to quit at 15. It took me another 15 years after that to actually quit smoking. I remember sitting in my therapist's office one day crying to her about how angry I was with myself about the fact that I was still smoking, and how badly I wanted to quit, and how hard I was trying.

"Why do you want to quit?" she asked me.

"Because," I told her, "smoking is so bad for you, it's disgusting, it's so lazy and gross. I just hate that I do it."

"What's the big deal?" she asked me. "If you wanna smoke, just smoke."

"But I don't want to! I hate it!"

"Seems like you're spending more time hating it and hating yourself for doing it than anything else. If you want to smoke, just smoke and stop trying to quit."

"But I'll die!"

"We all die! If you want to smoke, just smoke. No big deal!"

I left her office with an amazing sense of relief and happiness! I could smoke. I delightedly lit a cigarette as I drove home. And the next day I quit for good.

Why is that? Well, first off, I had a great desire to quit smoking, but I was very, very resistant to it. Once I was given the permission to smoke, the resistance was no longer there. When I thought that I could smoke, I wasn't grappling with the thoughts of, "I can never smoke again, how am I going to make it for the next three weeks? What about this party next weekend?" None of that was running through my head because I was allowed to smoke. In giving myself permission to smoke, I didn't have to deal with all the doubts and fears about quitting. Without those things in my way, quitting was much easier. It's often not the task that makes things difficult. It's the resistance to the task that is so hard to push through. One of the ways to work through resistance is to stop trying to work through it. When you come up against it, accept it. If you find that you are resistant to reading this book or doing this program, think of the reasons that you have decided to do it, and give yourself permission to stop whenever you want to, or to do it at your leisure. For example, rather than having to read the whole book at once, pick it up when you feel like it. Take a few months to get through it, or even a few years. If you don't want to do it in order, you just want to thumb through it and do the exercises that resonate for you, then do that. Sometimes, just allowing yourself to have autonomy and to have authority over your own decisions can be so liberating.

Going on a diet of course can be something that you become very resistant to because the diet itself has authority over you and your choices. It's easy to see where someone would rebel against that. That's often the reason why diets lead directly to binge eating.

Resistance is a normal reaction to change, so rather than fighting with it, and being swept away from what you are trying to achieve, embrace it and understand it. Eventually, you will find that the acceptance of the resistance itself will help you to flow forward with your recovery.

Your Inner Critic

Ultimately, in healing from Binge Eating Disorder, the goal is to be so in touch with your body, to love yourself and your body so much that you respect it, listen to it and get rid of the filter between mind and body. The filter is that part of you that comes between your wise mind and your body. Your wise mind is *the part of you that knows*. Not the part of you that fights your needs, not the part of you that beats yourself up, but the survivor in you, the part of you that loves you and wants you to live a full, healthy life and knows what you need in order to achieve that goal. Ideally, your body would send messages to your brain that it is time to eat and it would tell your brain what it needed. Unfortunately, when you have Binge Eating Disorder, there is something that intercepts that message and garbles it up. That's the part inside of you that tells you that you're fat, that part inside of you that tells you what you should and what you should not eat. The part of you that tells you that you are unsafe, unloved, defective... That is your inner critic – that nagging voice that lives inside your head and calls you names. It's the part inside of you that is incessantly criticizing, picking at you, always reminding you that there is something wrong with you, that you should be thinner, you should be eating less, that people think that you're fat, or ugly, or stupid, or that you said something dumb, that everyone should like you, that you should be a completely perfect person. It is always saying things like, "You should exercise more," or "You shouldn't have eaten so much," or "You should be skinnier..." or sometimes even worse things like, "You're a fat pig," or "You're stupid," or "You're dumb," or

"People hate you…" or "People will think that there's something wrong with you…"

Do you know that voice?

If this is familiar, you are intimately acquainted with your inner critic. The critic is your super-ego on speed. Your super-ego is the part of your psyche that is set up to keep you from acting on the impulses of your id, or your libidinal drives. Freud described it as "retaining the character of the father". So, basically, your super-ego is the internalized voice of the disciplinarian. Your super-ego keeps you from acting out on your dangerous urges.

When you suffer with an eating disorder or disordered eating the super-ego is overdeveloped and spins out of control. Rather than something that helps you create and maintain healthy boundaries, it becomes a structure that is set up to emotionally abuse you if you step outside of the rigid framework that you've created for yourself, even if you haven't ever been able to live up to the expectations or wants that you have set up. Some people have such out of control expectations for themselves that they become paralyzed and are never able to even attempt to reach those goals. This often sets up a cycle of self-loathing and self-abuse.

Why does the critic develop this way? There could be several reasons, or no reason at all. You might have had highly critical parents who only loved you when you did something right and punished you when you did something wrong. You might have parents who were very loving toward you but not very loving toward themselves. It's difficult to learn self-love when it's not modeled for you.

The critic tells you that there's something wrong with you, when there's probably nothing wrong with you. The critic tells you that other people are thinking that there's something wrong with you, which might or might not be true; either way there's nothing you can do about it, you can only really change your view of yourself.

As you begin to hear the critic without listening to it, you will find that it becomes a voice in the background that you can acknowledge without becoming a slave to it. As you travel further down your journey and learn how to love yourself, you will find yourself being able to challenge the critic. Eventually you will find that it has lost power over you and will find yourself feeling more joyous, and you sink into feeling comfortable with who you really are.

You might find that you are so enmeshed with the critic inside of you, that you are unable to separate yourself from that voice, the voice that feels like it is actually you, but really is not. It's the snotty, insecure teenage girl that lives inside of you who is constantly judging you, saying things like, "You're so fat, you're so ugly, you're so stupid, no one likes you…" blah blah blah. This voice isn't real. Though it feels like all of you, it isn't. It's just a small part of you that has taken over like a virus. This critic is not helpful. You might really believe that it is there to help you, that it will help you to be a better person, but it won't. Think about a child. Does a child feel good about herself and try harder when her parent tells her that she is a stupid, bad child? No, the child feels terribly about herself. She eventually acts out as a bad child because this is what is expected of her. But what if a child is loved and encouraged? She is then more likely to feel good about herself and achieve more in life. One of the ways to challenge your critic is to first notice it. When you feel yourself hearing things in your head like "fat, stupid, ugly… no one likes you," blah blah, the teenage girl mantra… first notice it, notice that this is not real, this is your critic. No one else is saying these things about you, just you are. And what if they are thinking these things about you? First off, they probably aren't, most people are too self-absorbed to think too much about other people. Chances are if they are thinking these things about you that they themselves are very self-critical as well. If they are having critical thoughts about you it doesn't matter. The only thoughts that can hurt you are your own. So having loving, peaceful thoughts about yourself will just feel better. To do this you must actively challenge those critical thoughts and then find your inner nurturer. So, when you're at a party or even just at the grocery store and you're looking down and feeling as though everyone is thinking bad thoughts about you, remember that it's actually you that are thinking these thoughts about yourself and imagining that everyone else is focused on you and having all of these mean thoughts about you. You might even have some empathy or a softening if you imagine that everyone else is sitting or standing there thinking about themselves and worrying about what others might be thinking of them. Notice that this is not real; everyone thinking bad things about you is not a fact. It's a belief that your critic has conjured up for you. Tell your critic to leave you alone. Take a deep breath, look up and smile at someone, anyone. If they don't smile back, find someone else to smile at. Try to get out from under your critic by connecting with other people. If love and peace and happiness are put out and mirrored back to you, your feelings will begin to transform. If you are submerged by your critic, you will feel trapped under its crushing weight and isolated by it, even if you're with a bunch of people. You can be trapped alone in your head with your critic only to find yourself angry, sad and lonely. Try really hard to offer love outward and let yourself receive it as well. In Step Twenty-One, I will show you more ways to escape from your critic.

Shame

One of the great components of Binge Eating Disorder is shame. Shame for bingeing, shame for the body that you're in, shame for doing things such as stealing and hiding food, eating out of the garbage pail, or lying about when or how much you ate.

Renowned shame researcher Brené Brown defines shame as "the intensely painful feeling or experience of believing we are flawed and therefore unworthy of acceptance and belonging." As a human being, you want to feel inherently valued and loved for who you are, not for what you do or for how you look. But when you hold shame you feel damaged at your very core, as though the essence of you is broken. And then, you either work constantly to do whatever you possibly can to change who you are to be a better or a different person, which turns into self-abuse; or you try to destroy the damaged person by making her into something different, something better, but that has the same outcome. You destroy yourself. The opposite of shame is self-acceptance. As you begin to accept who you are, you stop trying to destroy that person with bingeing, starvation, purging, excessive dieting, compulsive exercise, abusive self-talk, or other self-harming behaviors.

One of the most consistent side effects of eating disorders that I see is the overwhelming feeling of guilt and the deep sense of shame. Almost everyone with disordered eating has extreme guilt and shame issues. These issues aren't just limited to feeling guilty about the eating disorder or feeling ashamed because they have an eating disorder. There are nuances that weave through and perpetuate the eating disorder. Feeling guilty for eating, feeling ashamed of being a certain size, feeling ashamed for having 'no willpower' and then punishing oneself accordingly. This could be through purging, excessive exercise, restricting, or bingeing more. This could be through self-deprecation, name-calling, self-mutilation, isolation and other self-punishing behaviors. Those feelings permeate every part of your being. They're not always just: "I'm bad because I ate too much." They can also be, "I am bad therefore I don't deserve to eat," or "I am generally a bad or pathetic human being."

Food is not a moral issue. Foods themselves don't carry moral judgments. Eating a candy bar doesn't make you a bad person the same way as eating a head of lettuce doesn't make you virtuous, though so many people attach virtue to eating light.

Where having guilt is having the belief that you have done something wrong and feeling badly about it, shame is the overwhelming feeling that you are generally bad, worthless or unlovable. Some people try to overcome the pervasive shame feeling by dieting – they believe that if they are small, they will go unnoticed or not be open to scrutiny. Others try to avoid it by stuffing that feeling with food; they learn to hide under layers of pounds, helping to keep themselves hidden.

Shame begins when we are exposed to outside forces that tell us that there is something wrong with us, or treat us as though there is. This could be a parent, or a friend, or even a paradigm, religion, belief structure, a movement or a culture. A person who grows up as a minority in a close-minded town might be given messages by some people that there is something wrong with them, and grow up feeling shame. Someone born with a birthmark on her face might be teased by kids at school, or treated differently by teachers and therefore believe that she is defective, growing up feeling as though she must not do anything to draw attention to herself. She then makes her body as small as possible in order to become immune from being picked up.

Children who are emotionally, physically or sexually abused are taught that there is something wrong with them, that they must keep secrets, that they must be small and quiet. These children might try to make themselves as small as possible to hide, or as large as possible to be protected. The physically and emotionally abused child grows up believing that there is something wrong with them, that they are bad. The sexually abused child grows up feeling contaminated or infected. They believe that their worth is tied up in being a sexual object rather than a human being.

Healing from shame is about relearning your value. This does not mean making yourself more valuable or more worthy. You already are valuable and worthy. You are! This is about beginning to understand your value. Believing in your worth. The antidote to shame is acceptance. This means sharing your secret, finding safe people who love you unconditionally, and beginning to uncover your own worth. Healing is not about working on yourself or changing who you are. It's about becoming yourself, loving yourself and accepting the beautiful person who exists, who has always existed.

Chapter Five

The Inner Wars

There are several ongoing battles that occur for every disordered eater. The polarized thinking and habits that occur in binge eaters are an outward manifestation of the internal wars that are constantly being fought. So, in effect, when we have war with ourselves on the inside (internal conflict), we begin acting out our inner world outside of ourselves. Fritz Perls, who developed Gestalt Therapy, uses eating as a metaphor for the way we approach life. If that is true, then the paradox of binge eating would be well illustrated by the inner turmoil that plagues disordered eaters. Binge eaters fight these battles daily:

Battle between healthy self and unhealthy self.
Battle between healthy weight and unhealthy weight.
Battle between healthy mind and unhealthy mind.
Battle between healthy eating habits and unhealthy eating habits.
Battle between your own true body weight and society's perception of what an acceptable body should look like.
Battle between what your body actually looks like and what you believe your body should look like.
Battle between your wants and needs for yourselves and your family and friends' expectations of what you should be or do.
Battle between skinny and fat.
Battle between self-love and self-hatred.

Healthy Self vs. Unhealthy Self

Your healthy self doesn't just relate to your body; a healthy self is also a healthy self-image, as well as a healthy mind and spirit.

Though the belief is that everyone wants to be healthy, it's not necessarily true when it comes to eating and food issues. Being healthy would mean giving up the obsession. Giving up the obsession would mean the possibility of not being thin. Many disordered eaters tend to shy away from accepting a healthy self because that might mean giving up the dream of getting to their goal weight. It might even mean gaining more weight. This might seem counterintuitive; however, a large part of binge eating is driven by the same drive to be thin. When you obsess over your weight so much, food becomes your central focus. You might hold off on eating for as long as you possibly can by sending messages to yourself that you're fat, you don't deserve to eat and that you will continue to be until you lose weight. You might tell yourself that you won't be okay until you become thin. The critic continues to badger and bait you until you just need to take refuge in the one thing that brings comfort – food!

Healthy Mind vs. Unhealthy Mind

The goal in recovering from an eating disorder is to remove the filter between your mind and your body. The filter ignores your bodily cues for hunger and satiety. It tells you to eat when you're not hungry and tells you not to eat when you are. It also encourages you to eat or drink things that aren't going to be healthy for you, such as a Diet Coke or a cup of coffee to stave off hunger when your body really wants to be nourished at that moment. This filter, which contains your critic, is the unhealthy mind – the part that causes the eating disorder, or, as many people in recovery call it, "Ed". Calling it Ed personifies the eating disorder, which can help you think of it as something separate from yourself, something to battle, not something that is inherently a part of you. Ed tells you all sorts of things, like that you are fat or that you don't deserve to eat or that if you are hungry, that you have to distract yourself by doing different things. I had a patient who was so possessed by Ed that she would write things like "fat pig" in permanent marker on her arm to remind her not to eat.

This is clearly not a healthy mind. This is Ed, and it's often difficult to distinguish your healthy voice from your unhealthy eating disorder voice. Your eating disorder voice has no stock in your health and well-being. Your eating disorder voice is myopic. It has one goal in mind – which is either 'get skinny' or 'get more food' and usually it's both. That's the eye of the storm in this war; the internal paradox that is destroying you. It doesn't look at your whole body; it doesn't look at your health. It doesn't care; which is why when an eating disorder takes over, it ravages a body. It can become so pervasive and so overpowering that it doesn't allow any openings for healthy mind. Your mind is taken over by a cruel dictator who gives you instructions that you must follow without question. At this point, you begin blindly following the instructions without thought or consciousness. You've been possessed by the eating disorder. Several of my patients have described binge episodes as blackouts. They don't realize what they're doing until either they are halfway through a binge, and in some cases until it's over. This is the eating disorder taking over. This is where you need a proletariat uprising of epic proportions. Think of your healthy mind as 'the people'. They clearly need to band together and work hard to overthrow Ed, the evil dictator. Individually, they cannot do it. The dictator is too strong. However, a huge part of healing and getting your healthy mind strong is to enlist an army of support. Think of the supportive people in your life who you can enlist. If this is not an option, there are 12-step groups, online groups, group therapy for eating disorders, therapists, or you can even start your own peer support group for women going through similar issues.

Healthy Weight vs. Unhealthy Weight

Now, there's a pretty big problem with the concept of a healthy weight. First off, usually it's determined by an arbitrary height and weight chart or a BMI calculation. Some people just don't fall into those parameters.

At 5'2" inches, there are some women who would be very thin at 130 pounds, others who would be more voluptuous or full figured. For some people, being curvy or voluptuous is their healthy weight, and for some, being rail thin is their healthy weight. It's dependent on genetics, body frame, bone density, and body composition. You just can't base your weight on what's outside of you, like other people's weights or like charts and figures; when you do, that's when the trouble begins. This is an inside job and only you can find your healthy weight.

When you begin to listen to the wisdom of your body (more on learning how to do that later in the book), you will find a body size and shape that is pleasing to you. Your body doesn't want to be uncomfortably larger than it is meant to be. It doesn't want to be painfully skinny either, so as you begin to relearn your internal cues for hunger and satiety, your body will naturally land at its healthy weight. Your body's natural weight isn't necessarily the same weight as a Victoria's Secret model. It might be larger or smaller. However, your body does not deserve to suffer, to be made unhealthy because you believe that it is supposed to look different than it naturally does. Just as we can accept that people come in different heights, can't we accept that they have different frames and distribute weight differently?

Healthy Eating vs. Unhealthy Eating

What are healthy eating habits? Well, generally speaking, those could be three healthy meals a day or six light healthy meals a day, or 2 large meals a day. What is healthy is following your bodily cues for hunger and satiety. Eating when your body is beginning to feel hungry and stopping when you're feeling satiated.

However, in a person who has been dieting, bingeing, compulsive eating, fasting, starving or purging, those cues are distorted by urges to act out in the preceding behaviors. Thus, healthy eating and unhealthy eating are confused. Unhealthy eating tries really hard to win this battle. It does things like withhold food from you when you're hungry. It tries to fill you with things like water, Diet Coke or lettuce when your body needs a solid meal. It forces you to eat a box of cookies when all you really wanted or needed were a couple.

Healthy eating on the other hand allows you to enjoy one or two cookies when you want them. It gives you the ability to choose a cheeseburger or chicken breast or filet of fish when your body is craving extra protein. It will have you eat a big salad when you need some fiber or a banana or avocado when your body is craving potassium. Healthy eating is on the same team as healthy body. Unhealthy eating plays for unhealthy body. They love to fight with each other because the eating disorder doesn't care if you're healthy or not. Ed just wants to run your life. It is your responsibility to take your life back from him.

It's important to begin to recognize when Ed is in command. When he is steering the ship, it's crucial that you look for your healthy body/healthy mind and see if they can take over.

Your Natural Body Size vs. Society's Perception of What Your Size Should Be

Not one of the unfamiliar problems here is that the current archetype of the perfect female body is a woman who is shaped like a young child with large breasts. So, here we have a woman with gangly thin limbs, trim hips and thighs, a tiny waist and gigantic breasts. This body is, for the most part, not often achieved naturally. There are of course some people who are born with this body type. However, women come in all different shapes and sizes. Some are tall and skinny with flat bottoms and flat chests; some are short with round bottoms, full thighs and large breasts; some have flat chests with large thighs. Some are round; some are pear-shaped; some are curvy; some are more linear. Some have long torsos and short legs; some have long legs and short torsos, and on and on and on. There are as many different body shapes as there are people. Yet how is it that we then decide that there is one body shape that we are supposed to fit? And why is it that so many people hurt and torture their bodies to try to turn them into someone else's shape?

Partially I believe it is that so many people buy into this struggle because it's so important for human beings to feel accepted and acceptable. However, it will be impossible to believe that you are acceptable until you are able to accept yourself. No one else should have the power to dictate whether or not you are acceptable. So many people tend to project that power onto others, believing that they're not okay until other people think they're okay. The truth of the matter is, no one else is that concerned with your weight; they are too busy being concerned about their own lives. If they are spending their precious time judging your body shape, that's probably because they feel inept themselves, and are needing to judge and criticize others to feel good about themselves. It is much easier to push people down to feel elevated than to elevate one's own self. However, when one spends time judging and criticizing, they are still in the same place. They might *feel* better about themselves, but it is artificial. They have done nothing to better their self; they have just belittled other people so that they feel bigger.

We all have our own personal paths and dharma. It's important that you walk your path. Your path is different than others' just as your body size and shape has its own natural course. If you spend your time looking at other people's paths, you fail to see what's on yours. This is how to reject your life and abandon yourself. You become paralyzed and stop moving forward.

Your Body Weight vs. What You Think You Should Weigh

Again, your belief about what your body should look like might possibly be an arbitrary idea, not based in reality.

Tracy, a petite athlete, had the belief that she was supposed to weigh 118 pounds and that elusive number, that GOAL weight, became both her nemesis and her obsession. Though at 5'2", medically speaking, 118 pounds would have been a fine weight for her, Tracy's body was much happier at 130 pounds.

Beginning at age 15, she sought to reach that number. In high school, she was on the cross-country running team and was actively dieting, but still couldn't seem to lose those extra 12 pounds. During her first semester of college, she survived on nothing except one salad a day consisting of romaine lettuce and grilled chicken. By the time she went home for winter break, she was down to the coveted 118 pounds. However, being at home, she was confronted with the temptations and the comfort of all of her favorite foods. One night, just before Christmas, she succumbed to the pressure and binged until she could barely move. She justified this by vowing to go back on her romaine/grilled chicken plan the next day. Unfortunately, the next day, she was unable to do it. The seal had been broken and the binge continued for the remaining five weeks of her break. She returned to school 20 pounds heavier than when she'd left. This began Tracy's cycle. She would try to starve herself but, inevitably, the binge would take over.

Often, when people spend long periods of time restricting their food, their bodies become so afraid of starvation that survival mode kicks in. When this happens, they find that they are unable to do what they had previously done to lose weight. It feels as though the binge is taking over. The polarized thinking says, "This is the last time I will ever eat a cookie again, because tomorrow I can only eat romaine lettuce for the rest of my life; since I'm never going to eat them again, I might as well eat them all now."

Tracy was obsessed with food the whole time she was in college, not spending a whole lot of time on her studies, and alternating between starving and bingeing. However, her weight remained relatively stable, give or take a few pounds either way. Her body was fighting with her to remain at its natural weight and she was fighting back. In her junior year, she had to drop out of school because her eating disorder had completely taken over her life. She was unable to think about anything else other than food. All she did was exercise, restrict and binge. Her studies meant nothing to her. Her life revolved around the number 118.

And the years rolled on. By the time I met her, she was 25 years old. She looked lovely and seemed to be a perfect weight. However, she wanted me to help her get to 118 pounds. She said that she had around 15 pounds to lose, although she weighed herself daily and was running 5–6 miles every day without fail and she believed that if I could help her stop bingeing, that she would reach that weight. However, at the same time, Tracy believed that when she stopped bingeing, she could go back to her romaine/grilled chicken regimen that had worked for her briefly 7 years ago. I explained to her that if she was ever going to stop bingeing, she had to stop restricting as well. This was completely unacceptable to Tracy. She didn't want to let go of the idea that she could weigh 118 pounds. The problem was, she couldn't without being very sick. I explained to her that the last ten years of her life, the thousands of miles she logged running, all the lettuce, all the restricting, the bingeing, the obsessing, dropping out of school, all of it, she stayed within the same five-pound range up or down either way, and that this wasn't going to change. I asked her to do a few things to start.

1. Cut down her running to 3–4 days per week and no more than 45 minutes each run.
2. Either hide her scale, or bring it in to my office to hold for her.
3. Eat three square, healthy meals a day without restricting calories or carbohydrates.

I'd like to tell you that she agreed to try to work toward doing those things, in order to get a grip on her binge eating. However, she became very angry at my suggestions, refused to agree to anything like that and terminated therapy. She did not actually want me to help her to stop binge eating; she wanted me to support her eating disorder. She wanted me to fuel the obsession and help to perpetuate it. I was unwilling to do that.

The clutch of the arbitrary goal weight – that elusive number – can hold on with an excruciating grip. The number is not based in reality. It might be something on a height and weight chart, but it's not necessarily the weight that your body is comfortable at. If your body is truly healthy, it will fight against weight loss. A good part of this is accepting the natural weight that your body wants to be.

Your Wants and Needs for Yourself vs. Family and Friends' Expectations of You

One of the great personality consistencies that I find with people who are binge eaters is that they tend to worry much more about other people than they worry about themselves. They worry about what other people are thinking about them; they worry about whether or not people think that they are good people; whether or not people like them; whether or not people think that they are smart or stupid or fat or skinny, pretty or ugly. Generally, they spend endless days obsessing on what other people are thinking about them. They become absolute people pleasers completely sacrificing their own needs and doing whatever they can to take care of people around them. This becomes an intense negative feedback loop.

Christina grew up in a loving environment with two loving parents as well as an older sister whom she adored. Christina's mother Dora, though she loved her daughters very much, tended to criticize them as often as she hugged them. Dora's intentions were not to be overbearing or mean; she simply lived in fear of other people hurting her daughters. She thought that if they were perfect, then no one could hurt them. Dora's parents were also critical, but they were also both physically and emotionally abusive. Dora became incredibly placating, doing whatever she could possibly do to avoid abuse and criticism by her parents. As most abused children are, Dora became hypervigilant as an adult. She was constantly on alert, reading people's body language, presuming their motives and intuiting their needs. This was a survival mechanism that she developed as a child to keep herself safe from abuse. As a mother, although Dora was not abusive, she was petrified that her girls would be hurt by other people. In order to shelter them from this, she would constantly tell them that their hair was messy and to fix it, that they had gained weight and should go on a diet, that their hips swayed too much when they walked... Whatever she could criticize, she would. This, she believed, would keep her daughters safe. As you can imagine, this backfired. Christina's older sister became very rebellious. She was very promiscuous in high school. She left college due to a very serious drug addiction, which she has spent many years battling. Ten years later, she's still not completely recovered. Christina, however, went the opposite way. She became very compliant. She was so afraid of her mother's criticism that she did anything she possibly could to avoid it. Like Dora, she spent her days anticipating others' needs and completely sacrificed her own needs to take care of other people. As an adult, rather than speak up for her needs, she would go out of her way for everyone around her. She used food to stuff her feelings. Because she believed she was unable to have feelings or needs, she had to push them down with food. Christina was completely obsessed with what other people thought of her. If she walked down the street and heard people laughing, she was positive that they were laughing at her. She felt used in all of her friendships, as though people just used her for rides, to borrow money, to go out for meals, for babysitting, whatever it was. She obtained a martyr complex where she was grinning through her teeth, doing things for people constantly while resenting them at the same time. But she didn't know how to say no. She didn't understand that she could still have friends because she was a good person; she didn't understand that she was perfect, just by being who she was without having to meet everyone else's needs.

It was even worse for her in romantic relationships. When she became involved with a man, she became hypersensitive to his needs, completely rejecting her own. She became lost in trying to take care of a man at the expense of herself. Inevitably, none of these relationships worked because she wasn't actually there. After a few months, the men she was with not only felt smothered but they also felt bored being with a woman who had no sense of self. Her level of security was so low that she found she tried to achieve a sense of security by clinging to the men around her. She believed that would keep her grounded. However, what she was lacking was a deep sense of security within. If she had that, she would have been able to form a loving relationship with herself, which would then allow her to have a loving relationship with a man or even a friend without defining herself through their eyes. She was such a wonderful caretaker, but didn't know how to use those caretaking skills to care for herself. She was so used to her mother's criticism that she constantly saw herself through other people's eyes. She believed that she was whatever other people saw her to be. So, she did whatever she could to make people like her so that she could like herself. It didn't work though; she was so obsessed and believed that people were constantly thinking about how ugly she was, how fat she was, etcetera.

As we worked together, she began to realize that her belief that everyone was constantly judging her was a *cognitive distortion*. She came to understand that it was not only wrong, but also incredibly self-obsessed. She spent so much time making up and believing her fantasies about what everyone else was thinking that she was missing out on the world around her. As they say in Alcoholics Anonymous, "What other people think of you is none of your business." As she began to understand this, she found that she didn't need to spend so much time doing things for other people. She began to understand that she wasn't a martyr, but she was trying to control what other people thought of her. As she began to grasp the fact that she couldn't control other people's thoughts, she could only control her own, she began to become more comfortable with herself. She began to do exercises to help her quash her negative self-talk and begin to see herself in her own eyes. She decided to like what she saw. This was an active choice on her part. As she began to let go of her people pleasing, she began to feel less resentful. She found that she was bingeing less because she didn't have the need to stuff her feelings. As she learned how to say no to people, she began to learn how to say yes to herself. Saying no was very liberating. She did lose some friends. It's true that in many cases, when people begin to take care of themselves, to heal and recover, they often lose some people in their lives. However, this was okay with her. She kept many close friends and her relationships were enriched. People were finally seeing her, seeing who she really was rather than what she did for them, and people liked that! Those who were mostly using her left her life. Christina entered into a very serious relationship with a great guy. The relationship was completely reciprocal – they took care of each other. She tried her best to meet his needs, but did that without sacrificing her own. Because he loved her, he didn't want her to sacrifice her needs; he wanted to compromise and find a way where they could both live happily. This was the first healthy relationship that Christina was a part of. She knew that he loved her for her, even if she didn't feel like cooking one night, or taking off work to drive him to the airport, or doing his laundry. She knew that he loved HER. And because she wasn't so obsessed with trying to control his thoughts about her and his reactions and actions toward her, she began to see herself and enjoy herself in this relationship.

Here is a good rule of thumb. When someone asks you to do something, think about it before you say yes. If you don't want to do it, will you feel guilty if you don't? Will you feel resentful if you do? If the answer is yes, there is a good chance that you are rejecting your own needs to do this. It might be a good exercise to practice saying "no" and work with your own guilt rather than harboring resentment at someone because you have not set boundaries. This isn't to say that you should never make sacrifices for other people. Sometimes it's necessary. However, if you are constantly making sacrifices, you are losing yourself; and for many, the way to feel better about this is by treating themselves and comforting themselves with food.

Christina has been binge free for more than four years now and is continuing to have rewarding relationships with friends and her boyfriend.

Skinny vs. Fat

Yup, some people are skinny and some are fat. Some are thin and some are obese, some are stick thin and others are curvy. However, there is an unspoken rule that those who have the skinny genes are somehow blessed and those who have curvier or larger type builds have been cursed or are somehow inferior. It is suspected that people who are larger don't have the discipline or the willpower or the drive to be thin. Of course this is untrue. There are several very skinny people who never exercise and eat junk food constantly. There are also many larger people who are dedicated to healthy eating and exercise. Yet, we are still taught to look at skinny people as the quintessence of good health, discipline and purity. Fat people are thought to be hedonistic and lazy. There's something wrong with this. Especially as all the young skinny starlets continue to end up in rehab and have their pictures shot with them smoking and drinking excessively. Skinny is not good and Fat is not bad. Size, like food, doesn't have a moral value. It just is.

Self-love vs. Self-hatred

For some reason, it is not readily acceptable for people to love themselves unconditionally. For many there are certain rules and conditions that they put on themselves to deem themselves worthy of love, and that goes not just for self-love, but for allowing others to love them. Many disordered eaters set up rules about body size: "I can like myself when I reach xx pounds," or rules about food, "I can like myself if I eat no more than 1200 calories today," or dietary restrictions, "I can like myself if I give up sugar." There are even some organized groups that deem people to have a defect in character if they are unable to remain devoted to those rules or abstinent to the foods they shun for themselves.

Your love for yourself should not be conditional. That is a learned behavior, "I am only worthy of love when I..." Self-love is the only thing that will get you to the next level. Loving yourself will give you what you need to heal yourself. Hating yourself will do nothing but hurt you.

Chapter Six

Types of Binges

People are as different in the nuances of their disorder as they are in personality. Some people binge on cereal, others on bread, others on dried fruit, and others on ice cream and cookies. I had one patient who regularly prepared herself a rack of ribs and binged on that. However, there are a few main patterns to bingeing that we'll discuss.

Binge eating comes in two distinct patterns, binge eating with inappropriate compensatory behaviors and binge eating without compensatory behaviors. Compensatory behaviors are anything that you do to attempt to cancel out the binge. Such as starving, purging, or exercising. The following binge behaviors are the most common:

The Binge-Restrict Cycle

The binge-restrict cycle is usually what happens with the polarized (all or nothing) thinker. This is the person who starves all day and then binges at night. This is also the person who spends one day gorging and the next several days living on lemon juice and water. This occurs because the thinking is so rigid and so severe. Ally, a 25-year-old patient of mine, tried to maintain a zero-carbohydrate diet. Her daily menu consisted of water, Diet Coke, and cans of tuna. However, this lifestyle was nearly impossible to maintain. And because she was so inflexible about it, each time she failed at it, she would binge. For instance, one evening, she went to dinner with a friend. She ordered a burger without the bun and a vodka with club soda. After a couple of sips of her drink, Ally's control wavered a bit and she snagged a small roll from the breadbasket. After eating that one insignificant roll, she realized that she'd completely sabotaged her diet. She then polished off 3 more rolls, ordered a side of French fries to go with her burger and ate a gigantic hot fudge sundae for dessert. After she got home from her dinner, though she was so ashamed of herself, she realized that this was her last time to go hog wild as she would be back on the zero carb diet the next day. She ordered a pizza delivery and while she was waiting, she took a quick drive to the supermarket for more ice cream and some cookies. She spent the remainder of the evening binge eating. The next 3 days, she was back to eating perfectly on her zero carb diet. Again, though, it failed as one morning she was tempted by an orange. It didn't matter what the food was; if it had a carbohydrate in it, she felt like a failure.

Ally's binge-restrict cycle is quite common. This is one reason why severely restrictive diets don't tend to work. The inflexible nature of the diet contributes to the other side of the binge. The binge-restrict cycle can lead to Type 2 diabetes, electrolyte imbalances, heart attack, stroke, psychological distress, isolation – not being able to enjoy the activities that you once did, thyroid dysfunction, metabolic disorders and fertility issues among others.

The Binge-Purge Cycle

This is what we think of as Bulimia Nervosa. With the binge-purge cycle, the person either eats normally or restricts most of the day, and then eats large amounts of food and compensates for the binge by vomiting or taking laxatives. Purging with vomiting can result in internal bleeding and vomiting blood, spontaneous heart attack due to electrolyte imbalances, stomach ulcers, dental problems, vitamin and mineral deficiencies, hair loss, constipation and other digestive issues. Laxative abuse can also lead to a heart attack, as well as intestinal inflammation, constipation, systemic toxicity and dependence.

The Binge-Exercise Cycle

This is not healthy, moderate daily exercise. This is when someone eats a large amount of food and tries to work it off through excessive exercise. This is also referred to as compulsive exercise disorder or exercise bulimia.

A former patient of mine spent upwards of 3–4 hours per day at the gym, completely avoiding her friends, family, school, pretty much her whole life. Eventually a staff member who had noticed her obsessive behavior confronted her and encouraged her to get help. A body can only take so much.

Exercise bulimia can result in stress fractures, broken bones, sprains, muscle degeneration, bone density loss, heart attack, joint issues, overtraining syndrome, stress and anxiety over not being able to exercise and social isolation.

Non-Compensatory Binge

Most people who binge eat do so without compensating for it. This is usually eating normally and also bingeing without doing anything to 'get rid of it'. The bingeing can be occasional or frequent. This can sometimes lead to health issues such as obesity, Type 2 diabetes, heart disease, hypertension, stroke, gallstones, osteoarthritis and sleep apnea, as well as stress, anxiety, and depression.

Chapter Seven

Binge Eater Personality Types

You might find that you fit one of these profiles very well, or a few of these profiles, or you might even have traits of all of them.

The Perfectionist

If you fall into the perfectionist type, you probably believe on some level that you have to be perfect in order to be acceptable. You need a perfect body, perfect eating habits, flawless skin; you might believe that you always have to act perfect, always say and do the right thing, your house has to be perfectly clean, you have to have the perfect car, you just must be whatever you think perfection is. The problem is, of course, that nobody is perfect so in striving for perfection, failure is inevitable. Often, because of that, trying to be perfect becomes a frustrating letdown and a horrible blow to self-esteem. "I messed up, therefore I'm a failure, I suck, I'm a horrible person..." and descent into depression follows, which perpetuates further eating disorder behavior and other compulsive behaviors. You might not believe that you're a perfectionist because you seem to be the opposite, a total failure – this might be because you have such impossibly high standards for yourself that you feel absolutely paralyzed by the ridiculous amount of work you'd need to do to get to the place that you believe you should be. You can barely function in life because your belief of who you should be is so unattainable that you figure, "Why bother?" and live in a stuck place where you are unable to go forward with your life because you hate yourself so much for what you are not.

You also might be the type of perfectionist who does move forward through life with grace, speed and agility, but it's never enough. You always believe that you need to be doing more. You believe that when you get to a certain point, you will then be okay and like yourself. The problem is you never get to that point. You always want more for yourself. You are never allowed to like yourself and be okay with who you are. If you mess up, you punish yourself.

The perfectionist binge eater type usually has very rigid eating regimens and food plans. If they eat something off their plan, they wind up bingeing and figure they'll start all over again the next day. Alternately, they might punish themselves by purging or doing excruciating exercise.

The perfectionist often has the deep-rooted core belief that they are not good enough. They are extremely concerned with what other people think of them and believe somewhere that they can control what other people think of them by being thin and perfect. Of course, as you know, it's always beyond your control as to what other people think of you. If you are kind and hold yourself with integrity, people have no reason not to like you. However, if they don't, it has nothing to do with you. You just cannot spend time trying to make people like you. It is a poor use of your time as it is impossible to please everyone. Just ask any US president. No matter how popular you are, millions of people hate you. There's not much you can do about it. Just continuing to do the things that make you like and respect yourself is the way to feel more comfortable with imperfection. You bring contentment and peace to yourself by giving yourself validation, rather than doing a million things to get it from someone outside yourself. You can't be perfect, but you can aim to be a good person by trying to be compassionate and kind to those around you while striving toward goals with gentle loving support from yourself. That is the kind of perfection all human beings are capable of and the kind that will make the world a gentler, happier place to be in.

The Emotional Eater

If you are an emotional eater, food and mood are intrinsically linked. When you are feeling sad, you grab food. When you are feeling agitated, you go for food. When you feel anxious, you go for food. You even go for food when you are feeling happy or celebratory. The emotional eater is unsure as to how to manage her feelings. Most emotional eaters are very sensitive people whose feelings are felt so strongly that they can be overwhelming. Food helps to dull the sense of being overwhelmed.

If you are an emotional eater, you usually label your emotions as positive or negative. For instance, sad, angry or scared are bad emotions, but if you are happy, that is good. When you notice a 'bad' feeling, you try to stuff it down with food. Learning how to accept and sit with challenging feelings is the beginning of healing from emotional eating. Food used to be the antidote to feeling badly. But as you begin to incorporate mindfulness and sit with, talk about, write about and process your feelings, you won't need an antidote; you will be able to manage them.

The Stress Eater

If you are a stress eater, you use food to deal with such life challenges as bills, debt, unemployment, taxes, illness and other stressful everyday occurrences. You can become so overwhelmed by everything that you have to take care of that you wind up munching to calm the anxiety that comes with having to deal with these things. Unfortunately, after using food to deal with stress, the original stressor is still there. So now, the bills have yet to be paid, and you have the additional discomfort, guilt and shame from the binge.

Using mindfulness, meditation and deep breathing as part of a stress management program will help you to heal from stress eating.

The Student

The student can be a high school, college or graduate student. Schoolwork is overwhelming and procrastination ensues. Late nights up doing homework lead to late night pizzas. Fear of poor grades, anxiety over getting papers done, all you can eat cafeterias, parties with lots of alcohol, hangover binges... College students are perhaps the most at risk for binge eating. All the ingredients are there, such as the brand-new autonomy to choose what and when you eat coupled with the all-you-can-eat/open-all-night cafeteria while dealing with the anxiety and stress of being away from home and dealing with highly charged interpersonal relationships and unstructured time.

Students have to learn how to balance their lives by prioritizing studying, sleep, exercise and healthy eating.

The Binge Eater in Denial

If you are a binge eater in denial, you might be in a bit of a fog about your binge eating issues. The binge eater in denial is unable to see the choices that she's making. She believes that she is a normal, healthy eater, despite evidence to the contrary such as failing health or rising weight and of course frequent binge episodes. For instance, she'll claim to herself and to those around her that she's eating healthy or that she never ever eats anything 'bad'. Then, in front of people when she eats something she deems inappropriate, she'll make grandiose statements like: "I never, ever, ever eat like this." Mostly she eats in secret, almost as if in a blackout. Often she doesn't even remember her binges. They can actually take over and feel as if they just happen.

There is a lot of compulsivity around food because the level of consciousness is not there. It's challenging to make choices about food because there is such a great deal of denial. Not just about food, but about emotions as well. This will make it challenging to exercise restraint or boundaries around food. She will eat even if she isn't hungry if there is food in front of her. It's hard for her to notice what she's doing because she is barely there. It's almost as if she's just not in control of her body or her actions. She has very little consciousness around her food intake. She often binges in her car, going from takeout restaurant to takeout restaurant in a daze, without noticing what she's doing.

This is obviously very challenging because the binge eater in denial feels completely out of control. People will tell her to eat less and exercise more. More than anything she wants to do this, but she feels completely unable. The goal here is to begin by raising consciousness of both your feelings and your behaviors. Eventually, as you begin to become aware of what you're feeling and why you're choosing to eat, you are able to gain control and thus are able to choose how you want to be with food.

The Constant Dieter

If you are a constant dieter, you are probably always trying the next new thing to lose weight. You pore over fashion and fitness magazines and diet books. You know enough about nutrition to have a PhD in it. You have a ton of exercise equipment in the house, some used, some barely used; you know the calorie or carbohydrate count of most foods without looking it up. You've tried every diet and know them all. You've lost thousands of pounds but put them back on and taken them back off.

The constant dieter is very black and white in her thinking. If she is on a diet and 'slips' by eating perhaps a croissant or a muffin, she believes that she messed up the whole day, and figures that tomorrow is another day when she has to restart, so she might as well binge for the rest of the night.

Giving up dieting and learning intuitive eating is paramount to healing the constant dieter binge eater.

The Binge Drinker Eater

The binge drinker eater uses alcohol to keep her from eating. She will get home at night, and rather than eat dinner she'll try to satisfy her need for food by downing a few cocktails. She'll go to a party after not eating the whole day and just drink wine. Of course this backfires as the alcohol makes it less likely that she will be able to control her eating and will begin to eat with reckless abandon. If she winds up not eating, she will probably get very drunk from the lack of food and have a binge the next day to help her get through the hangover. In this case, alcohol is being used as a way to deal with food cravings. It goes without saying that substituting dinner for a bottle of wine is unsafe.

Of course the answer to this is to always have a full meal before beginning to drink alcohol. But if you believe you have a drinking problem, you need to tackle that with treatment in order to find a place of recovery. Alcoholism and eating disorders go together more often than you'd think. If you think you might have a problem with alcohol, I'd recommend both talking to a therapist who specializes in recovery and attending at least six Alcoholics Anonymous meetings before you make a decision about whether or not you need treatment.

The Pavlov Binge Eater

If you are a Pavlov binge eater, you always eat a certain food as a response to external stimuli. For example, you always have to have popcorn or nachos at the movies, cheese fries at the mall, pastries with your 4pm latté, and eggnog at Christmas. Rather than thinking about what you want or what you need, you'll eat something because of a learned behavior to eat a certain food at a certain time.

Letting go of this behavior is about beginning to associate memories with the actual memory, not with the food. For instance, going to the theater is about the entertainment, the mall is for shopping and your 4pm latté is about taking a break from work. It's also about remembering that there will always be eggnog at Christmas, there will always be another tub of popcorn. Just because it's there, doesn't mean you need to eat it.

It's not going away.

The Nighttime Binge Eater

If you are a nighttime binge eater, you are probably 'good' all day. You might either eat regular healthy meals or you might restrict all day long. Either way, you find yourself bingeing in the evenings. People often binge at night as a response to the stress of the day, or as a way to fill a void of loneliness and boredom, or as a way to unwind, shut down and relax. Some studies have shown that night eaters have serotonin imbalances that lead them to use food medicinally.

Beginning to understand what you actually need in the evenings and learning how to give that to yourself is the way to let go of nighttime binge eating.

You might identify with one of these subtypes of binge eaters, or a few, or have some aspect of all of these. You might have something going on that I didn't even mention. However, I can pretty much guarantee that whatever it is that you're doing with food, you're not the only one, and there is a way to heal.

This isn't About Anything Else, I Just Want to Lose Weight and I Want to Lose It Now!

You might just feel that you can't identify with any of this, that you just want to stop bingeing, be able to stick to your diet, and lose weight quickly. That need for instant satisfaction is paramount in our culture. But it's a task of Sisyphean proportions. Sisyphus, a character in Greek mythology, was a king who was punished by having the task of rolling a giant boulder up a hill. As soon as he got this boulder to the top of the hill, it would roll back down, and he had to traipse back down, get the boulder and roll it back up the hill again. This cycle was to repeat itself for all of eternity. That's sort of what happens with fad diets. You get on an extreme food and exercise plan in order to quickly reduce your waist size – how many times have you tried to lose 10 pounds in 2 weeks or something similar? You NEED immediate satisfaction and you demand it. This is the other side of compulsivity, not compulsive eating, but compulsive dieting. You want what you want when you want it, whether it's cake or a size 4 body. But, life tries to maintain a homeostasis – an evenness or stability. When you compulsively restrict, it comes out the other side when the compulsive binge happens. When you lose weight quickly, you put it back on just as quick, or even quicker.

Slow weight loss is not only sustainable, but it teaches you about your body. It helps you to begin to understand what your body needs and how to get it there. Your life has been mapped around bingeing and restricting. All of this quickness, this compulsivity, is a huge part of the cause of binge eating and it's a quick fix. "I don't want to feel my feelings so I'm going to stuff them with food. I can't deal with what I'm feeling, I'm going to run away from them by over-exercising. I can't deal with what I'm feeling, so I'm going to restrict my food and thus cut off what I'm feeling. I can't deal with my husband so I'm going to obsess on what I'm eating or not eating. I don't know what to do with my career so I'm going to obsess on my body. I'm going to obsess on these things because it's the one thing that I can control since everything outside of me feels so out of control…"

Slowly learning your body and letting go of the need to control gives you so much more information into who you are. It allows you to take time out to think about your needs, not just your food needs, but your physical, spiritual and psychological needs.

This is all about slowing down and sitting with your uncomfortable feelings of stress, sadness, anxiety, or whatever it is that you don't want to feel. As you increase your tolerance for uncomfortable feelings, you stop eating to make them go away. You don't need to focus on a diet; you can focus on your life because your feelings, even the really hard ones, become more tolerable.

I know that everyone wants to lose 10 pounds in 2 weeks or

less. And of course that's possible, but at the same time it's dangerous. Very few people who do this maintain that loss. You have to do something very drastic to reduce your weight so dramatically so quickly. As soon as you begin to eat normally again, you instantly put the weight back on. Staying on a drastic diet long-term is not feasible. It invariably turns into an eating disorder and causes a multitude of health problems. Quick weight loss, while desirable, is a fantasy that is left just as a fantasy. When you are eating three very healthy meals a day, without bingeing and allowing yourself the occasional treat, your body will naturally fall to its healthy and natural weight. This might take two months and it might take two years. However, learning at this very moment to give up your bingeing might be worth the time. I've seen people on the cycle of losing several pounds in a very short time and regaining them again in a very short time, back and forth for years on end. They become chronic dieters. Because their plan worked once, they always believe that it will work again, so they try that one diet that worked 20 years ago, and continue to fail. However, if that really worked, people would only have to diet once ever. In the name of quick weight loss, people wind up in a cycle that lasts a lifetime, just like Sisyphus. They say, "But this time I'm not going to gain it back." It almost never works.

Chapter Eight

Getting Started

Choosing to Love Your Body

You get one body. That's it. This is the body you are born with, and unless you choose to spend a great deal of time and money on plastic surgery, this is the body you have. When you feed your body not just with healthy foods, but with loving thoughts, your body will repay you 100-fold. Hating your body is superfluous time and energy. It is also painful. You are less likely to take care of something you hate. If you love your body, you will be more likely to treat it with love and respect by feeding it three healthy meals a day, giving it water, taking your vitamins, and treating yourself with respect. If you hate your body, you are more likely to hurt it. You are more likely to punish it with unhealthy food, or hurt it with compulsive exercise or by depriving it of nourishment. Body love isn't easy, especially when women have been taught for so long to hate their bodies, but it is possible.

Finding Support

Before beginning your steps, make sure that you have a support network in place. A support network is any person or group of persons whom you feel safe with. Because these steps can be so emotionally charged, it's important to have your safety checks in place. These support people are those who you can do the exercises with, or just those who you can talk to about what you're going through as you do the exercises. For many of you, your instinct will be to just read the book and go at it alone. While this is possible, I really want you to consider the fact that eating disorder behaviors are usually acted out alone and in isolation. Many people become very isolated in their disorder, sitting home alone and bingeing, going to sleep, feeling sad and alone, feeling powerless and then beginning the same cycle again alone. Because eating disorders thrive in isolation, they are also defeated in company. It is crucial to your recovery to create your own team of support to help you beat this. The forces acting against you and outside of you are immense. You need to create your own army to fight these forces.

In thinking about your support network, safety is something to really ponder. How do you know if you feel safe with someone? A safe person might feel safe to talk to about certain things but not about others. Find someone who feels safe to talk to about your food issues. A safe person is someone who won't judge or criticize you, who won't give you advice or dieting tips. A safe person listens without judgment. A safe person does not try to tell you how to fix yourself. A safe person is not in competition with you. Many women have girlfriends with whom they've had a relationship based on dieting together for years. Often these women have an unvoiced competition going on with each other. These are probably not the safe people whom you want to choose to support you with your process. If you can't think of any safe people in your life, perhaps a therapist or counselor can be helpful for you during this time. You might also find comfort in a 12-step group such as Overeaters Anonymous or Eating Disorders Anonymous. There are so many people who struggle with similar issues. Sharing and understanding others' experiences, strengths and hope helps to make you stronger and the disorder weaker. There might be someone in your life who you just have to coach to be a safe person. You can let them know that you are going through this process and you need someone to listen to you, but not to give you advice or to criticize. Many people will be receptive to this and almost relieved. You might even form your own support group of two or three other people who want to do the steps together. Whatever you choose, it's important not to do it all alone. Binge Eating is a disease of secrecy; but like a monster in the dark, when you shine the light on it, the monster disappears.

Change is Hard

If it were easy, we wouldn't have so much trouble adjusting to new habits or changing old ones. We are constantly fighting against the current. Think of your life as a rolling river, and you are in an inner tube floating down that stream. You might not be enjoying it, you might want to redirect yourself, but the easiest thing to do is to be carried by the river. In order to change, you have to fight against the flow. Healing from binge eating is an amount of work. We constantly fight against change.

Unconsciously, we want to maintain the homeostasis in order to allow our condition to stay constant and stable. Our binge eating serves a purpose and when we take the binge eating away, other systems must change. In order to allow for that to happen, something must intercept from the outside to help that change happen. Going through these steps are the outside stimulus that will help change to be more viable. It might not be easy, but the rewards on the other side are great – being free of binge eating, feeling safe in your body, feeling safe around food and feeling safe with your emotions.

Mentally and Emotionally Preparing

Healing from Binge Eating Disorder involves changing your way of thinking from using things outside of yourself to make your life better, to making internal shifts by understanding that you have everything you need inside of you to be okay... even if you think you don't. It's about strengthening the wise self inside of you to enable you to draw from it in times of stress or pain, rather than looking outside of yourself for an answer.

Binge eating is using food as an answer to many of life's challenges and disappointments. Like people who abuse drugs and alcohol, people can begin to use food to self-medicate. Whereas some people have a drink or two if they're having a bad day, others use it to cope with every single aspect of life. What they thought was the solution has become the problem. And of course it builds on itself and only gets worse. The pathological abuse of food to deal with life becomes the medicine that the binge eater begins to abuse. What once worked, now becomes distressful, painful and the main focus or problem in their life.

As compulsive eating and compulsive dieting mix together to create the soup of Binge Eating Disorder, many people get stuck in a molasses swamp of beliefs that if they were thin, their lives would be perfect. Healing from Binge Eating Disorder isn't about becoming thin. It's about finding more productive and healthy ways to manage the stress of life and to find healthy ways of coping with the pain and the emotions that cause you to binge eat.

If a symptom of your binge eating is being at a body weight that's not right or is unhealthy for your body, weight loss or gain will be a natural part of your recovery process. If you choose emotional strength, healing, and inner peace as your goal, your body will also settle into a place that feels peaceful and easy to be at because you are choosing to treat yourself with love, compassion and respect.

Exercise: Finding Your Wise Mind – *Journal Opportunity* and *Meditation Time*

Your wise mind is your gut feeling, it is when you know something to be true in your bones; *everyone* has a wise mind. It might be so quiet that you think it does not exist, but it exists in almost all of us. Your wise mind is the part of you that intuitively understands the truth. It is your intuition mixed with your knowledge of information that feels right and healthy. Your wise mind exists to help you to know truly what is the best decision for you on a deep, heart level. When you find your wise mind and learn to listen to it in order to make decisions or gain information about how you feel, you will find that you are more peaceful and confident about your decisions. You will have much less self-doubt and anxiety and more confidence. In eating disorders, the voice of the wise mind is often drowned out by the voice of Ed. When you find your wise mind, you will trudge through the violent ocean of voices and come to find the quiet peaceful voice of your truth. You will tune out the loud unyielding eating disorder voice and only listen to your wise mind. Ed might not stop talking, you might still hear him; however, you can choose not to listen and not to engage with that voice, but instead to truly listen to the voice that is wise and nurturing. To find your wise mind, follow these steps:

1. Close your eyes, put your hand on your chest and find your heartbeat. Just allow yourself to be with the beating of your heart as you find calmness in the rhythm of your beating heart.

2. In your mind's eye, locate your inner core. The inner core is the strength inside of you, the light that guides you on a daily basis. It might be very dim, barely shining, but it is there and the more you focus on it, the stronger it becomes.

3. Notice what it looks like, and notice what it feels like inside of you.

4. How do you feel as you focus on this part of yourself?

5. Ask to speak to the wise self that lives inside your inner core. Just wait as she emerges. You might see your wise self as you, except strong, glowing, effervescent, ethereal, and illuminated. You might see your wise self as your 200-year-old self. You might see your wise self as someone you know who has passed away or someone who is still alive that you look up to. You might even see your wise self as an animal. Just wait to see who emerges for you and then spend some time there with your wise self. Your wise mind is part of your wise self.

6. Ask your wise self what it is that you need right now, and just listen. Don't try to force an answer, just be silent, continue to breathe, and listen.
7. Draw a picture of your inner core and your wise self to remind yourself visually of what you always have inside of you.

Whenever you are sad, in trouble, in pain, stressed out, put your hand on your chest, take a few deep breaths, visualize the picture you drew and ask: "What is it that I need?" If you are quiet and you listen, you will most likely find the solution inside of yourself.

You will begin to realize that food, dieting, all those external solutions are not actually solutions; that what you need is what you already have inside of you.

It will probably be tough to find an answer at first; you might not hear any answers even the first several times, but continue doing this exercise. Just like building muscle strength, building core strength takes time, patience, faith and dedication. As you continue, you will find a deep internal strength that will guide you through the worst of times. It's simple and it is always there for you.

Part Two

A Step-by-Step Guide

To Healing From Binge Eating

How to Do the Steps:

These steps are not meant to do just once. As you grow and evolve, your feelings will change dramatically. You can do the steps several different times at different periods in your life. Doing these steps in a journal will help you to see your progress and understand the way your feelings change and how your recovery has evolved over time. It is best to do these steps one at a time. My recommendation would be to do one each week or every couple of weeks so that you can really process them and take time to master them.

Step One – Create Purpose

The very first step in achieving any goal is having an under-standing why you want to achieve this goal. All goals need to be backed up and motivated by purpose. Motivation and purpose is what moves you toward your goal. Without it, your goal will be very difficult, if not impossible to achieve.

Quitting binge eating might be difficult, but anything worth doing takes discipline. Make a promise to yourself that you won't quit when it gets hard. When it gets hard, that's the good stuff, that's what exercises your intention muscles. The more you work through the difficulty, the easier it gets. If you gave up whenever things became difficult, you would have never learned to read or write, or even to walk or talk.

It is so easy to quit when things become difficult. It is not easy to keep going, but it is worth it. If you quit and resume your binge eating, what will happen? Binge eating might feel better and easier in the moment, but, as most people know, it feels awful the moment after. And, of course if you quit, you can always come back to it. It's not the end of your journey.

Creating purpose will help you to keep going when you want to quit. If you remember the reason that you are choosing to work on this, you will find that it is easier for you to pick yourself up when you choose to quit.

Exercise One: Going Back in Time – *Journal Opportunity*

If you could go back 15 years into the past, what would you tell your younger self? What lessons have you learned and what kind of changes would you make? Write a letter to your younger self, telling yourself exactly what you wish that you had known then.

Writing Prompt:
Dear Self, I am coming to you from 15 years in the future to give you some valuable information:

Now, close your eyes and try to imagine yourself 15 years in the future. If you were to continue traveling down the trajectory that you are on now, what kind of advice would your 15-year-older self give your present self:

Writing Prompt:
1. *Dear Self, if you continue to follow the path that you are currently on, this is where your life will be:*
2. *Here are some suggestions for ways to continue on your path:*

Exercise Two: Why Should I Stop Binge Eating? – Journal Opportunity

1. List every reason to quit binge eating:
2. Now, make a list of reasons not to quit binge eating – this list is important. It helps you to understand your saboteurs. If there were absolutely no reason to continue it, you would have stopped a long time ago:
3. Looking back at these letters and these lists, what do you notice?
4. Do your reasons for quitting binge eating outweigh your reasons for holding onto it?
5. Now, check out your reasons for not quitting binge eating. Look and see if you can challenge any of them:

Check out the following example:

I don't want to quit binge eating because it's too hard:

Challenge Statement: It is hard, that's true, but as I work to transform this habit, it will get easier. It takes time, dedication, and discipline, and I have the strength and the resources to do it. I know that I can't be perfect at something right off the bat; I have to practice. Even if it doesn't happen immediately, I am willing to practice this skill in order to give up binge eating.

I don't want to quit binge eating because it's the only thing that makes me feel better when I am sad:

Challenge Statement: Sometimes it makes me feel better, but oftentimes it makes me feel worse. I also know that it's not true that the only thing that makes me feel better is binge eating. Sometimes talking on the phone to a friend helps, other times taking a walk outside, and still other times, renting a movie and watching it and zoning out in other non-food related ways can help.

What are **your** reasons?

I don't want to quit binge eating because:

Challenge Statement: Try to come up with a challenge statement for every reason that you have not to quit binge eating.

Exercise Three: *Art Project!*

For this you will need either index cards, drawing paper, construction paper, or you can even use clay or sculpting materials.

Go back to your reasons for wanting to quit binge eating. Write down each of those reasons on one side of the card or paper, and on the other side draw a picture illustrating what that means to you. You can even mold or conceptualize your reasons. For instance, if you write, "I want to feel peaceful around food," draw a picture of yourself feeling peaceful or create a picture of what peace and calmness looks like to you. Or if you write, "I want to go places that I normally avoid because of food," draw a picture of yourself out in the world, enjoying your life and doing the things that you want to do.

Step Two – Learn Intuitive Eating

The first part of integrating intuitive eating is vowing to give up dieting. I know I know I know. No one wants to give up dieting. We always think – "but I know that if I can do this right this time, I'll be perfect – finally." Or, "but I've dieted before and I was happy…" Or, whatever other reasons we give ourselves to diet. Honestly though, how many times have you dieted? Where has it gotten you? Where are you now? Are there people who can diet successfully? Perhaps there are. However, this isn't a diet book. This is a book for those who are binge eating and can't stop. Dieting is the other side of binge eating, and in order to find balance between the two, you must halt both behaviors. The goal is to find a middle ground.

I am defining dieting here as the deliberate act of restricting food in order to achieve weight loss. This includes low fat diets, low carbohydrate diets, low calorie diets, fasting, cleansing, and counting calories.

Does that scare you? Giving up dieting can be an incredibly frightening proposition to many people. For many it means giving up control. Actually though, dieting is a false sense of control. Many people start dieting when their lives feel out of control. It can lead to a sense of comfort, a belief that you have gained control of your life. You believe that you have control, but if you are binge eating you have a complete loss of control. The diet controls you and the food controls you, and then the binge controls you. Many people fear that when they give up dieting they will spiral out of control, and their body will expand out of control. The truth is though, that when you give up dieting, you can actually begin to stop listening to the constraints of a diet and start listening to your body.

Giving up dieting doesn't mean giving in to compulsive eating. It doesn't mean giving in to a free-for-all. It's about giving your body what it needs when it needs it. It's about giving yourself enough of the right foods to feed your body and eventually allowing yourself to occasionally have treats and previously forbidden foods that you would binge on in the past.

As you begin to feed yourself nurturing foods, as you begin to give your body what it needs when it needs it, your body will settle into its natural weight, which is a place that will be very pleasing to you. As we continue on with the book and the exercises, I will teach you to get in touch with the true needs of your body. You will begin to hear the voices of what your body needs rather than the voices of the dieter inside of you. The dieter convinces you to deny what your body needs, it rebels against the needs of your body; then the voice of the binger comes along and rebels against the dieter, trying so hard to get you what you need and often going overboard. The voice of the binger rebels against the voice of the dieter. And then, a vicious battle of dieting and bingeing erupts inside of you. You are literally being pulled into and controlled by a huge internal conflict. After you let go of that dieter inside of you, the conflict disappears and you have more space for the part of you that wants to be healthy and happy.

So go ahead and throw away your bathroom scale. Make a ritual out of it. Bring it to the dump, destroy it, vow that you won't weigh yourself unless you are at the doctor's office and she or he shouldn't even tell you your weight. You don't need an unsophisticated piece of machinery that spits out an arbitrary number to dictate how you're supposed to feel about yourself. No more morning weigh-ins, no more gym weigh-ins, no more weekly weigh-ins. Let go of having to know how much you weigh in order to know how you're supposed to feel. You are in charge now. You get to know how you feel by waking up and actually letting yourself feel.

I understand how this can be confusing: on one hand, the whole world is encouraging all different kinds of diets, yet a small contingent are telling you not to diet.

It's crucial for your long-term health and well-being to reframe the concept of dieting to lose weight to the idea of going toward health to improve your quality of life. Your body is your most valuable possession and therefore it deserves to be cared for impeccably. This doesn't mean spending hours each day at the gym and polishing your muscles and kissing your biceps in the mirror. This does not mean spending money on plastic surgery or Botox or liposuction desperately trying to change what you have. This is about embracing what you already have and taking really good care of it. This is about health, vitality, physical and emotional strength and well-being.

If somehow you had possession of an original Picasso, would you paint over it to make it look like an Andy Warhol? Or would you make sure to get it insured, keep it out of sunlight, store it in a climate-controlled environment, and really truly allow yourself to enjoy it? Taking care of it will keep it beautiful for a very long time, despite how much it ages. In fact, age enhances its beauty. It's the same thing with your body. Rather than trying to change it into something different, rather than disliking it the way it currently is, let yourself love it, no matter what size and shape it is. Your body deserves love no matter what it looks like. It's your body, the only one you got. So take care of it. Feed it healthy food, don't feed it too much and don't feed it too little. Give it healthy amounts of fruits and vegetables and limit the amount of processed foods that you put in it. Exercise it, stretch it, wash it, floss your teeth, drink your water, be kind to it, rest it, give it adequate amounts of sleep, take it outdoors to get fresh air and sunlight, bring it into nature, be grateful to it for whatever it gives to you, limit alcohol, tobacco, diet sodas, and other 'foods' made with chemicals, but don't freak out if you eat them every once in a while, relax your mind, listen to music, dance, be kind to yourself and to others.

When you choose to go toward health rather than going on a

diet and actively trying to lose weight, you will find more peace and happiness than you will when you are actively looking for it from a scale. When you take care of your body and your mind in a deliberate and loving way, you will find that your body weight naturally finds its right place. This isn't a diet; this is thinking about the rest of your life and your body in a positive way, and strengthening it for the long haul!

Exercise One: Exploring Your Feelings About Diets – *Journal Opportunity*

Think about what is coming up for you around the ideas of giving up dieting.

Example:

If I give up dieting I am afraid that:
I will gain so much weight that I won't be able to get out of bed. I am afraid that I will gain so much weight that no one will want to talk to me and my partner won't be attracted to me. I am afraid that I will lose my job and all of my friends, my husband will divorce me, no one will want to be with me and I'll be completely alone.

This makes me feel:
This makes me feel anxious. I am also angry that I am being asked to do this. This seems stupid and impossible.

What are the possible benefits of giving up dieting?
If I give up dieting, I might find that I have more fun when I go out. I might stop avoiding places that I've been avoiding and people who I've been avoiding. If I give up dieting, I might find that I can allow myself more of the kinds of food that I've been denying myself for so many years – except for when I'm bingeing. I might find that I feel more peaceful more of the time and less anxious around food.

I now feel:

A little calmer. I am still nervous, but I am willing to try giving up dieting for a few months and follow the protocol in this book. I am a little doubtful, yet I am hopeful. I'm willing to try anything at this point.

Now try answering these questions on your own, thinking about your own feelings:

1. If I give up dieting, I am afraid that:
2. This makes me feel:
3. What are the possible benefits of giving up dieting?
4. I now feel:

Exercise Two: How Has Dieting Impacted Your Life? – *Journal Opportunity*

This might help you to think more deeply about the cost/benefit analysis of giving up dieting. Ponder and answer the following questions.

1. How long have you been dieting?
2. What are the various types of diets you have tried?
3. What kinds of short-term results have these diets yielded?
4. What kinds of long-term results have these diets yielded?
5. What has your life been like as a result of these diets?
6. How would your life be different if dieting and food were not your focus?
7. If you weren't dieting, what kinds of things would you be able to do that you currently feel you cannot?
8. What kinds of places do you currently avoid because of your obsession with dieting, food and body image?
9. What would your life be like if you could do the things that you are currently avoiding?
10. What function does dieting serve for you?

11. How do you feel that dieting benefits you?
12. How do you feel that dieting hurts you?
13. What would it be like if you could do the things you have been avoiding without having to think about food, dieting or your body?

When it comes to dieting, the holding on is what is so hard, the letting go – *the surrender* – is easy.

Exercise Three: Weight Loss without Dieting

The whole world is telling you to diet and I am telling you to immediately stop dieting.

But what if you have a great deal of weight to lose? Please ponder these questions. First off, how do you know that you need to lose weight? Is it because you believe that you weigh too much, or is it because you believe that your weight is negatively impacting your health or your quality of life? Are you unable to enjoy your life because your weight is stopping you, or are your beliefs about your weight stopping you? There are some people who, at 5'5" and 145 pounds, believe that they need to lose weight and their weight becomes an issue for them. However, it's not really their weight, it's their thoughts about their weight. Could that be you? Is it your thoughts about your weight that lead you to binge or is it your actual weight? If it's your thoughts about your weight, please continue reading and working through the steps to help you begin to feel some comfort in your skin.

Of course I understand that you might be one of the people reading this book who is very heavy and your life has become challenging. You might be unable to do everyday things comfortably, like take a bath, sit in a restaurant booth, have sexual relationships and many, many other enjoyable things in life. Dieting must seem like the only solution out there. But I want you to reconsider that. How far has dieting gotten you? Oh

I know that you might have lost a great deal of weight on a diet once or even several times, and there's a part of you that thinks, "If I could just do that low carb diet again, if I could just stick to 1500 calories again, just like I did last time, I'd lose all this weight." But I'm asking you to reframe your thinking here. Rather than thinking about losing weight, think about gaining health. Your body is your most valuable possession and therefore it deserves to be cared for impeccably.

When you let go of dieting, you incorporate intuitive eating. Intuitive eating doesn't mean eating a whole pan of brownies when you want to. If you want a brownie, you think to yourself, "Will this trigger a binge, or will I be able to eat one in a healthy way?" If you intuitively know that right now baking brownies is not a good idea for your recovery, then you need to let go of it for now, not forever.

The following intuitive eating steps that we will be going into in more detail throughout the book will help your weight to normalize:

Always Eat When You are Hungry. This is challenging for someone with Binge Eating Disorder because, sometimes, real hunger can become confused with wanting and needing other things (emotional hunger). Later on in the book, we will learn how to distinguish the two.

Stop When You are Satisfied. You don't have to eat until you are full. Eat slowly and mindfully. Listen for physical cues that tell you that you are not hungry any longer. Stop in the middle of a meal and ask yourself how hungry you are, how much more food you need, how the food tastes and how you are feeling. Many people eat until they are full or until they can't eat any more. You should definitely not leave a meal hungry. But if you can let yourself stop before you get full, your body will readjust to smaller portions allowing for weight loss.

There is a Confucian teaching that is known as Hara Hachi Bu, which instructs people to eat until they are 80% full. This is practiced by the Okinawans in Japan, who, incidentally have the highest average lifespan, 29% of the population lives to be 100. Try to go for 80% done. If you fail, that's okay. Don't restrict your next meal; just remember that you still have your next meal to try again. You won't get it right at the beginning; it takes practice to figure out what 80% is. The idea is to stop eating right before you are full. You can experiment by stopping your meal in the middle and asking yourself how you're feeling. If you are satisfied, you can put your fork down for five minutes, take a food pause. If you are not, eat half of what's left on your plate and check in again. The key here is checking in with your body constantly. Eventually this becomes second nature and you will find yourself finishing your meals before you're full, even without all those check ins.

Enjoy Your Food. Eat slowly, don't rush through your meals. Avoid eating standing up in front of the refrigerator, or while driving, or while lying down, or while in bed, or while walking, or in front of the television. Sit down and make a ritual out of each meal, even if the meal is just a smoothie, or a power bar on the go. Take time to enjoy what you put into your body.

Don't Stuff Your Feelings with Food. Part of using this book is learning how to comfort and nurture yourself without using food. Anger, sadness, anxiety, loneliness and boredom are all normal feelings. They're not good, and they're not bad. They just are. But, those feelings are *hard* to sit with and eating will just make them go away – quickly! But, as you know, it won't fix any problems associated with these feelings. It might temporarily soothe you, or numb you, but the problem will still be there after you've binged, and you will feel worse.

Respect Your Body. As you learn to give your body love and respect, you will find that you begin to feel more of who you are and better about that person.

Exercise with Love. Find a way to move your body that you enjoy. Yoga, Pilates, walking, jogging, swimming, dancing, any way that you enjoy moving your body will help you to find body love.

Step Three – What's Behind the Urge to Binge Eat?

Sometimes, the short-term gain of a habit can override the long-term gain of quitting the habit.

For example, your thinking could be, "If I eat this quart of ice cream right now, it will help me to feel better." That might be true; however, this is the time to begin to slow down and think about what will happen after you eat that quart of ice cream. "If I eat that quart of ice cream tonight, I will feel better and be able to get some sleep. However, I will wake up in the morning in a fog, feeling sick and uncomfortable. I will also be angry at myself. I might not want to get out of bed. I might skip work or I might not meet up with my friends the way I was supposed to because I'm feeling so bad about myself. That might result in me spending the whole day at home alone and bingeing..."

Although there is currently a great deal of emphasis on creating healing by living in the moment, and being in the now, this is very different than being compulsive. For example, if you are living in the now, you are being incredibly mindful of your thoughts, feelings, and needs. You are not trying to avoid them or push them away. When you are bingeing, you are giving in to an urge or a craving. You might think that this is what's happening in the moment, but actually the urge to binge is about avoiding what's happening in the moment. As you consciously let your mind slow down, you are able to stop to allow yourself to make decisions about what you really want to do. Have you ever felt like you woke up in the middle of the binge? That you didn't really plan it, that it just happened without your consent? This is the opposite of living in the moment. This is actually denying the moment, doing something to shut out the moment. The moment then rebounds and accentuates itself. If you are feeling lonely and you binge to shut out that feeling, you will feel lonelier after the binge. You are probably bingeing because you are feeling a feeling that is uncomfortable to you, whether it is boredom, anxiety, sadness, loneliness, fear, stress, anger, or any other feeling that is challenging to feel. The irony is, the last thing you need when you are feeling badly is to make yourself feel worse with the self-flagellation that often comes from bingeing. At this point, you need understanding, self-love and attention. Binge eating is actually a signal that you are trying to take care of yourself emotionally. However, you might not know how to, so you binge in order to make yourself feel better and then you wind up feeling worse. What a vicious roundabout that we can get trapped in!

Exercise: Understanding Short-Term Gains vs. Long-Term Consequences – *Journal Opportunity*

This exercise is designed to help you to understand why you binge eat, and what you hope to gain from it.

Short-Term Gains: What are some short-term gains that you get from binge eating?

Examples:

> *If I binge eat right now, I will not feel so lonely.*
> *If I binge eat right now, I will not be sitting here obsessing about going to the store or going into the refrigerator or picking up the phone to order food.*
> *If I binge eat right now, I will stop feeling so anxious or angry about something that recently happened.*
> *If I binge eat right now, I can stop lying here having this argument with myself.*

Write down some of your short-term gains from binge eating.

> *If I binge eat right now...*

Long-Term Consequences: What are some of the longer-term consequences of binge eating? Think about how you will feel and what happens when you binge eat.

Examples:

> *If I binge eat, my stomach will hurt.*
>
> *If I binge eat, I will fall asleep without getting anything done tonight.*
>
> *If I binge eat, I will feel become overly full and bloated and feel uncomfortable in my body.*
>
> *If I binge eat, I will be angry with myself.*

What are some of your longer-term consequences of binge eating? Write down some of your own consequences of binge eating:

> *If I binge eat...*

Step Four – Figuring Out Your Binge Triggers and How to Defeat Them

Binge triggers can be either emotional, physical, situational or a particular kind of food. At the beginning of recovery, it's not easy to understand what your triggers are. That's because when you are triggered to binge, it feels as though the binge is automatic. However, as you become aware of what your triggers are, you will have the consciousness to make the choice as to whether or not you are going to binge.

Emotional Triggers

Many people who binge eat have difficulty identifying feelings. Whenever they are feeling something, rather than identifying and tending to the feeling, they turn to food. For example, you get a bill in the mail from your cell phone company telling you that you owe them $1400 for calls that you never made and it sends you right to the kitchen or nearest bakery. What is it that you're actually feeling? Stressed? Angry? Helpless? Sometimes a trigger can be something as innocuous as seeing a commercial on TV, perhaps of two people getting married. It might make you feel sad or lonely if you are not in a relationship but wish you were. These are the kinds of small events that can easily set off a binge.

Feelings are a barometer of what is going on around you. They help you to identify a situation as safe or unsafe. They help you to understand your mental state at the time.

Physical Triggers

Not all binge triggers are emotional. Some are physical. Some people find that after eating out, they will binge. This might be because they feel too full. The feeling of being too full can be uncomfortable and then trigger a binge. This seems paradoxical, but it is a common occurrence amongst binge eaters. Many binge eaters have lots of issues with shame around food and the urge to lose weight. Feeling too full might create a sense of shame, which perpetuates the bingeing cycle. At the opposite end of the spectrum, feeling too hungry can lead to a binge. This is for more obvious reasons. Sometimes, the dieter will restrict food to a dangerous extent. At this point, their body is so hungry that it takes over, trying to get as much nutrients as it possibly can while the control centers are not watching. Some people equate this to sneak eating.

Maggie, a patient of mine who had been struggling with Binge Eating Disorder since she was 12 years old, had always been larger than her very petite sister. At a young age, her mother put her on a diet and she wasn't allowed to eat the same things as her sister did. If the family had pizza for dinner, Maggie was served a boiled chicken breast with peas and carrots. No dessert for her, no treats. Maggie's mother could not understand why she wasn't losing weight. She took her to countless doctors and nutritionists. Maggie wasn't losing any weight because she was sneak eating. She had to be perfect while her mother watched her eat; but alone, she would dive in to Twinkies, candy bars, and any other kinds of junk food she could get her hands on. As an adult, she would eat 'perfectly' for most of the day and in front of people. But in private, she would ingest huge amounts of cake and candies. She hated herself for it, but couldn't stop. As soon as Maggie began to actually allow herself to eat the foods that she had been denying herself, she found that her binge eating decreased. As she began to forgive herself for not being perfect and not eating perfect and chose to allow other people to see that she wasn't perfect, she began to recover.

Another physical binge trigger is being tired. I've heard many women in my practice talk about needing a nap, but bingeing instead. Partly they are hoping that the food will wake them up. Sometimes, they are just so tired that they can't bring themselves to nap, and other times, they just don't have time. They use sugary foods to give themselves a lift.

Yet another binge trigger is having a headache, being physically sick or injured, having either a food or alcohol hangover, or being in pain. You might feel totally powerless against whatever ailment is occurring in your body, so you soothe yourself with food.

Situational Triggers

There are also places that cause people to binge, for instance their cars, airports, their parents' houses, parties, or any other situation that can be anxiety provoking. Car binges are super common for people dealing with Binge Eating Disorder. I've heard many stories of people intentionally car bingeing, by going from takeout restaurant to takeout restaurant and planning their day or evening around their binges, to more unintentional binges, like picking up groceries and bingeing on them on the way home.

Binge eating while traveling is also common. Airport layovers are recipes for a binge because:

1. Traveling is stressful and binge eating is a stress relief.
2. You are bored and it's a way to fight boredom.
3. Although you are traveling among several thousands of people, if you are traveling alone, you are in a city where nobody knows you and this can feel very isolated and anonymous and secretive.
4. There is a bounty of fast foods and 'forbidden foods' in a relatively small radius.
5. You might be going home to see your family.

Going home to your family can also be a recipe for a binge. Even if you love your family and they're very supportive, it's still challenging to be home when you're working toward recovery.

Your internal roadmap, the way you negotiated life, was created in this environment. When you are outside of the environment, it's a bit easier to change and revamp that roadmap. When you are back in, your default settings can be reactivated.

Classical Conditioning

Part of learning to trust your body is becoming aware of how things outside of your body influence you. Though bingeing is often a response to deeply felt emotions, not all binges are an emotional response; some are due to external stimulus.

In the late 1800s, Ivan Pavlov, a Russian psychologist and physician, learned about classical conditioning while investigating the gastric functioning of dogs. During his research, Pavlov noticed that not only did the dogs begin to salivate when they were given meat, they began to salivate at just the sight of the lab technician who normally fed them. Pavlov hypothesized that if he provided a certain stimulus at the same time as he provided food, the dogs would learn to associate food with that particular stimulus and they would produce saliva with just the association of the food. In order to prove his theory, Pavlov rang a bell when he fed his dogs. They then knew that the bell indicated food was coming. After a few repetitions, the dogs started to salivate in response to the bell. This came to be known as classic conditioning or a Pavlovian response.

People learn to associate food with a particular stimulus. For instance, they'll be at a movie theater and feel that they need popcorn or candy; or they'll associate driving to work in the morning with a donut and coffee; or Sunday mornings will always lead to pancakes or bagels. Most of us are not as simple as dogs; however, we can easily have behavioral and even physiological responses to certain stimuli. How have you been classically conditioned to eat? Do you expect cake every time you go to your grandmother's house? Do you always stop for pizza on your way home from a movie? Does your mouth begin to water (like the salivating dogs) when you see a commercial for a restaurant you love? When you become conscious of those common catalysts, it is easier to make decisions based on what your body needs than what you are conditioned to eat.

For as long as she could remember, Elena's grandmother always had a giant crystal bowl of M&Ms on her coffee table. As a little girl, Elena would run to the table and eat M&Ms. As she grew up, whenever she spoke to her grandma on the phone, she would suddenly get cravings for and buy M&Ms despite the fact that she did not usually eat candy. When she was 33, Elena's grandmother passed away. She spent several months bingeing on M&Ms. She went through several large bags each day, pouring them into a large crystal bowl that she kept on her desk at work. When she came in to see me, she talked about how she had been bingeing since losing her grandmother and wanted support around her grieving process so that she could actually feel her feelings and not stuff them with food. However, as she began to talk more about her grandmother and her memories of being in her home and feeling warm and safe, she began to realize that the M&Ms weren't just there to help her to alleviate the pain, but also to help her feel close to her grandmother again. She actually had the warmth and nurturing feeling from eating M&Ms that she got from being at her grandmother's house. Not only was Grandma's house equated with M&Ms, but M&Ms were equated to Grandma's house. When she began to realize that she was trying to replace the warm feelings of being with her grandma, she was able to replace those M&Ms with something more helpful. She put old pictures of herself and her grandmother up in her cubicle at work and kept a blanket from her grandmother's house at home in her bed to remind her of Grandma and help her to feel warm and safe.

Just being aware of these responses to stimuli can help you to change up your routine. For example, if you know that you binge on pastries every day on your way home from work, try taking a different route home, or carpool/walk with someone. Do you start bingeing as soon as you get home? Change your routine and take a shower or bath the first thing when you arrive home. Just breaking up your routine can be immensely helpful in changing your behavior.

Having triggers is normal. We all have triggers that set off behaviors that we don't like; it's part of being human. One of the wonderful things about self-exploration is beginning to understand what kinds of things trigger specific behavior so that you can make a plan to conquer that behavior before it happens. Hallelujah for being blessed enough to get older and really learn to know yourself.

Finding out why and when you binge is one of the most important steps to conquering this behavior. Having knowledge of yourself and awareness of why you carry out the behaviors that you do is a step to healing.

Begin by using this alternative action log. When you feel the urge to binge, write down what the trigger was, what you want to do, what the consequences are and what else you can do.

Exercise One: Create an Alternative Action Log

You can either create your own Alternative Action Log, use the one in Appendix F, or download one from the website.

When you feel the urge to binge, sit down with your Alternative Action Log and answer the following questions:

1. What Kind of Trigger was this, emotional, physical or situational?
2. Describe What Happened:
3. Feelings: (What am I feeling about it?) If you are unsure about what feelings are connected to the triggers, look at the feelings list in this appendix to see if you can identify what you are feeling.
4. Short-Term Solution: (What do I want to do in the short-

term to make me feel better?)

5. Long-Term Consequence: (How will that make me feel later, or tomorrow?)

6. Alternative Behavior: (What else can I do to make myself feel better?)

Although this log is used to help keep you from bingeing, go back and write in it, even if you have already binged. This will help you to understand more about what you were feeling in the moment. Notice what happened on the days that you binged. Were you trying to study for an exam? Did you get into a fight with your kids or your parents or your partner? Were you just plain bored? As you begin to understand what emotional triggers cause you to binge, you can prepare for them. You can create plans to stop a binge before it starts when you are in a potentially triggering situation. For example, your history of Alternative Action Logs shows you that you often binge after you get back from visiting your parents. You then realize that this is a danger zone for you, so you begin to make plans to sabotage the binge rather than allowing the stimulus to sabotage you. Such as, "I know that I'm going to have dinner with my parents tonight. My mother will comment on my weight and I'll be so hungry because I never let myself eat in front of her and I'll be so upset after dinner that I will stop at the store and get binge food. I have a plan. I'm going to bring a supportive friend with me to dinner, that way, if Mom criticizes, I have someone to be with afterwards to help me feel better instead of food."

Exercise Two: Create a "Do Something Different" List

As I said before, when you are binge eating, the last thing that you need is a pejorative dictator yelling at you and telling you that you are bad or that there is something wrong with you. What you need is care and compassion. Binge eating is a coping mechanism. The goal here is to learn new ways to deal with painful or challenging emotions, that don't involve stuffing your feelings down with food.

There are several ways to learn to be more gentle, loving and kind with yourself. There are also several different ways for you to give yourself a boost when you are feeling low that doesn't involve self-abuse. Later in the book, we will discuss internal coping mechanisms and ways to deal with challenging feelings. But right now, let's just figure out and incorporate some external alternative coping mechanisms to replace binge eating.

Write out a list of things that you can do to nurture yourself instead of binge eating. This is called a "Do Something Different List".

List as many alternatives to binge eating as you can think of. Begin by pondering what you would like to achieve by binge eating. Then think of something different that will help you achieve a similar feeling. Take that list, and perhaps paste it onto a beautiful, inspirational drawing and post it in a place where you will need it the most. For example, here is a list that my eating disorder group compiled together.

Do Something Different

1. Get out of your home and take a walk if it is safe to do so
2. Download music
3. Dance
4. Do crossword puzzles
5. Call a friend, a family member or a support person
6. Go to a bookstore
7. *Acknowledge your feelings and try to sit with them
8. Think about how you want to feel later – allow yourself to see your decision through to the end
9. Visualize something positive, like your life without an eating disorder
10. *Go to a support group meeting online or in person

11. Take a bath or a shower
12. Brush and floss your teeth
13. Light candles or incense
14. Lie down and rest or go to sleep if tired
15. Read a book
16. Write a letter/e-mail
17. Go through old letters or e-mails that make you feel better
18. Go through magazines and create a collage or vision board
19. Take out some art supplies and paint or draw
20. Do crafts
21. Do scrapbooking
22. Knit or teach yourself to knit or to sew
23. Go to church/synagogue
24. Watch a DVD or go out to the movies
25. Clean
26. Breathe/meditate/stretch/do yoga
27. Bring food to homeless people in your neighborhood or to a local shelter
28. Volunteer or research volunteer opportunities
29. Go through your to-do list and begin to cross things off
30. Have a spa day in your home. Give yourself a hot oil treatment, manicure, pedicure and facial.
31. Go out and get a manicure. You can't eat with wet nails!

What are some things that help *you* feel good about yourself or help you feel warm and happy? Continue this list on your own.

*Acknowledge your feelings and try to sit with them – this is discussed more in depth in Step Eleven.

*Go to a support group meeting online or in person: There are several free support groups for people who have issues with binge overeating. You can check for your local Overeaters Anonymous chapter by going to OA.org or, you can attend a meeting online or on the phone by going to http://www.oa.org/

meetings/find-a-meeting-online.php.

You can also form your own support group using the principles of this book to do so.

Exercise Three: Understanding Your Classical Conditioning – *Journal Opportunity*

1. Do you notice patterns about when you overeat or binge?
2. Are there certain routines where you habitually overeat or binge? For example, right when you come home from work/school, or after going out at night?
3. What are some ways that you can break up your routine in the times that you typically binge?

As you bring consciousness to your automatic responses, you will find that it is your choice. You have the ability to make the choices that you want to make about what and when you want to eat.

Step Five – Self-Monitoring

What? Another food journal? NOOOOOOOOOOOOOO... If you've ever been in any kind of recovery or on a diet before, you know about keeping a food journal. This is a form of self-monitoring and accountability to self. It gives you a sense of power and control and a responsibility to your self. In this food journal, you will not be counting calories, or points or carbohydrates. You will be keeping track of your feelings as they relate to your food. This is helpful because it allows you to understand how different foods affect your mood and how your mood affects what you decide to eat.

Start by just watching yourself. This isn't about trying to change anything yet; it's about becoming aware of your habits. This food and mood log actually helps you to become more honest with yourself about food.

By monitoring your food intake and being brutally honest with yourself, you can begin to analyze your behaviors and how they correlate not only with your moods but how your behaviors build on themselves. It's wise to monitor throughout the process of recovery, but if you can manage for two weeks, you will uncover a lot of important information about yourself. Continued self-discovery is another benefit of the recovery process.

This is an example of a food and mood log that Elizabeth, a former client of mine, kept.

If we analyze the food and mood log opposite we can discover a lot by asking the following questions:

What physical symptoms triggered a binge?
What emotional symptoms triggered a binge?
What could she have done differently to avoid a binge?

DATE, TIME AND PLACE	HOW DID YOU FEEL PHYSICALLY BEFORE YOU ATE?	HOW DID YOU FEEL EMOTIONALLY BEFORE YOU ATE?	DESCRIBE YOUR LEVEL OF HUNGER BEFORE YOU ATE:	DESCRIBE WHAT YOU ATE INCLUDING SERVING SIZE:	HOW DID YOU FEEL PHYSICALLY AFTER YOU ATE?	HOW DID YOU FEEL EMOTIONALLY AFTER YOU ATE?	DESCRIBE YOUR LEVEL OF HUNGER AFTER YOU ATE:
9:00am (office)	Tired	Anxious, I'm just at work and have a huge presentation that I'm not prepared for.	I'm not hungry, just an anxious stomach.	2 cups of coffee with cream and sugar	Jittery and amped up	I was still very anxious	I didn't feel hungry at all, I was just too scared to be hungry.
11:30am (office)	Exhausted	Really upset, my presentation didn't go well. I just want to hide. I'm ashamed.	I'm starved, but lunch isn't for another hour.	2 Danishes and 1 pack of cookies from the vending machine, another coffee	Sluggish and tired. Kind of greasy.	Sad, down-trodden, ashamed of having eaten the sugary food. I'm angry at myself for being unprepared and angry at myself for what I ate.	I'm actually still hungry, despite the high sugar, high fat, high calorific value.
12:30pm (office)	Still tired	Feeling hopeless about work. Don't want to be at this job anymore.	I'm really hungry.	One Diet Coke and two cups of coffee	Jittery, tired, and a little out of body.	Proud of myself for skipping lunch to compensate for the calories that I ate after the presentation.	I'm pretty hungry.

DATE, TIME AND PLACE	HOW DID YOU FEEL PHYSICALLY BEFORE YOU ATE?	HOW DID YOU FEEL EMOTIONALLY BEFORE YOU ATE?	DESCRIBE YOUR LEVEL OF HUNGER BEFORE YOU ATE:	DESCRIBE WHAT YOU ATE INCLUDING SERVING SIZE:	HOW DID YOU FEEL PHYSICALLY AFTER YOU ATE?	HOW DID YOU FEEL EMOTIONALLY AFTER YOU ATE?	DESCRIBE YOUR LEVEL OF HUNGER AFTER YOU ATE:
7:00pm (home)	Feeling exhausted. Have a bad headache	Anxious, happy to be home from work. Don't want to go in tomorrow.	I'm hungry but I don't want to eat.	One glass of water, 3 ibuprofen, 2 glasses of wine	Kind of drunk, exhausted and hungry.	Proud of myself for skipping dinner, still have the rest of the night ahead of me. Don't know what to do, I'm anxious about how to deal with the rest of the night.	I'm so hungry.
8:30pm	Exhausted, light-headed, still have a headache despite taking ibuprofen.	Depressed, lonely and uncomfortable.	I'm really hungry but I'm too tired to cook and there's no food in the house and I don't want to go shopping.	I drink another 2 glasses of wine, and then I decide to order a pizza. I plan on eating only one slice, but I wind up eating the whole pie.	I'm bloated, full, my stomach hurts and I'm so, so tired, and kind of drunk.	Uncomfortable, depressed and regretful. Lonely, and I hate myself for bingeing again.	I am uncomfortably full.

Looking at this food and mood log, what can you tell about Elizabeth? Clearly she was tired, hungry, anxious and depressed. Being too hungry triggered binges for her. Her first binge came in the morning. First off, she was exhausted; she hadn't slept enough the night before because she was anxious about the presentation that she had to make at work. And she left for work having not eaten anything; she was hungry. After her morning sugar binge, she felt so angry with herself that she avoided food for nine hours. She tried to use alcohol and caffeine to prevent her from eating, but in the end, her hunger won out and she ate a whole pizza. Her only food for the day was wine, coffee, Diet Coke, Danishes, cookies and pizza. Continual days of eating like that can lead to severe malnourishment. It's true that people can be both obese and malnourished at the same time.

There was obviously a lot going on emotionally for Elizabeth. She was unhappy with her job and her eating issues were feeling completely out of hand. She woke up in the morning very, very anxious about this big presentation that she had to do. Rather than skipping breakfast and just downing coffee, it would have been in her best interest to wake up a bit early and force herself to eat a light breakfast, something that she could have easily digested, yet something hearty enough to get her started on the right foot. She could have had a couple of eggs and a slice of toast or a piece of fruit and cheese or even a bowl of high protein/high fiber cereal, something that would allow her to focus and keep her satiated. Being sated in that way would have allowed her to take a moment to think about what she actually needed at 11:30 after her meeting was over. She probably didn't need to eat two Danishes and cookies and more coffee. She might have needed a bit more food, or she might have needed to get out of the office and talk to a supportive person about the presentation. She was clearly upset. She dealt with it by first stuffing her feelings with food, then by asserting power by restricting food and thus redirecting all the pain she had onto herself. She punished herself for whatever went wrong. She should have had a healthy meal at lunchtime rather than using caffeine to keep her from eating. She wasn't doing her body any favors by filling it with chemicals. She was avoiding food, but also avoiding what was going on for her at work; notice how that parallels. By the time she got home, she was exhausted. Her body was run-down by lack of nutrition and possibly lack of sleep. Had she eaten a healthy lunch, she might have been better equipped to shop and prepare herself a healthy dinner. But that didn't work either. She chose to drink instead of eat which was a poor choice which begat more poor choices. In this case, fatigue, headache, anxiety and extreme hunger were the triggers that caused Elizabeth to binge eat. By analyzing her behavior, she was able to understand what it was that created these binges. She knew she had to deal with the job situation as well as her anxiety, but she also had to relearn how to eat like a normal person. Restructuring her days around regular meals was incredibly helpful for her. That kind of structure created more space for her to understand her feelings and deal with them without abusing food.

Exercise One: Keep a Food and Mood Log

Begin to keep a food and mood log. You can find it in Appendix F or online.

In analyzing your food and mood log, answer the following questions:

1. What physical symptoms triggered disordered eating?
2. What emotional symptoms triggered disordered eating?
3. What could you have done differently to avoid a binge?
4. What patterns do you notice?
5. How many hours do you go between meals?
6. How do you feel when you're hungry?
7. How often do you let yourself get hungry?

8. What ways could you have taken care of yourself without using food?

Exercise Two: Face Your Trigger Foods

Create a list of trigger foods, foods that you notice you weren't able to stop eating after you started, or foods that brought on a binge of other foods. You might notice that your trigger food is something as innocuous as garbanzo beans. This isn't to judge, it is an honest 'noticing' of where you need support.

When you monitor for a week or two without making any changes, you will begin to better understand yourself and your motivations around food as well as your trigger foods, your trigger situations, your trigger emotions and your physical triggers. Once you do this, you deepen your understanding of what you need to help yourself recover.

Step Six – Making Your Home a Safe Zone

Now that you know what particular foods trigger you, support your recovery by getting them out of your space. Getting rid of trigger foods can be challenging, unrealistic and impossible for many people. For those who live with roommates, parents, children, spouses or partners, this might be very unrealistic. For those who live by themselves or with supportive family members or roommates, this will be much easier.

Clearing out your kitchen basically involves making your home into a war-free zone. At this point, you clear out all the foods that you know you have binged on. This includes healthy foods that you binge on. Anna, a self-professed health freak, had to clear her home of blue chips, hummus, dried mango, and macadamia nuts because she found that if she kept these snacks in the house, she would binge on them.

Clearing your kitchen out of binge foods doesn't mean that you are restricting; it means that you are making your home a safe haven, a place where you don't have to suffer with your anxiety about bingeing. This is a controversial practice. Some eating disorder professionals don't believe in clearing the home of triggers with the belief that the world is full of triggers. Learning to deal with them without giving in to them is what will heal you. I agree. However, I also believe that in early recovery, you can make it as easy on yourself as possible. This means creating a safe space. This does not mean that you can never have these foods in your house again; it is just in the early part of your recovery while you are trying to get a hold on your bingeing. If you were recovering from alcoholism, you wouldn't dare have a bottle of vodka in your freezer. The same holds true for your trigger foods.

Exercise: Cleaning Shop

Go through your list of foods that you are likely to binge on or foods that you have binged on. Ask a supportive person to come over and go through your cabinets and refrigerator with you. Get rid of all of those foods. Give them to your friend to get rid of for you.

If you live with a partner or spouse, you might need to sit down with them and explain to them what you're going through. You might need the assistance of a couples counselor. This is important. If you were an alcoholic, it would be crucial that your partner didn't bring alcohol into the house while you were going through recovery. Think of trigger foods like alcohol. You will feel more comfortable if they are not easily accessible.

As you go on in your process, you might begin to learn about different trigger foods that you never would have thought that you'd binge on. For instance, one woman in my practice discovered that she couldn't keep raw, unsalted pumpkin seeds in her home. If she did, she'd eat as many as she could and even if she finished them all, the binge momentum had been started and she'd continue with whatever she could get her hands on.

Once you've cleared the house of binge foods, vow not to bring any binge foods home and declare your house a binge-free zone. This is not a forever thing, but for now, in the early parts of recovery, you want to keep yourself safe. Just as a recovering alcoholic wouldn't spend time in a bar or keep bottles of gin in his or her home, you don't have to have your triggers constantly confronting you either.

Step Seven – What Should I Be Eating?

There are several different books that will tell what to eat and what not to eat. You should definitely do your own research and self-experimentation to decide what foods work for your body and give you the most energy and health. It's always a matter of slowing down and finding what feels right. This is where mindfulness and intuitive eating comes in.

In general, when you are recovering from an eating disorder, you want to begin to change your view of food from something to fear to something that is nurturing and life affirming, something that gives you strength, energy and vitality – the opposite of what your eating disorder does.

Optimally, if you can aim to have much of your diet made up of whole, unprocessed foods, you are in good shape. This is simply food that's in its purest form, and does not come in a package or have any added sugar, salt, preservatives or other added ingredients. An apple, a piece of meat or fish, fresh vegetables, and unprocessed grains are all considered whole foods. Processed foods would be anything in a box or a package, anything that is made in a factory rather than grown on a farm, anything that uses multiple ingredients and chemicals, such as candy, soda, processed meats, ice cream, frozen entrees, macaroni & cheese from a box, really anything that can sit on a shelf for a long time without going bad. Of course it's okay to eat these things in moderation but, when the bulk of your food comes from whole foods, that's where you get the most nutritional value.

As you most probably know, there are three macronutrients: protein, carbohydrates, and fat.

Carbohydrates are made of sugars and supply energy to your cells. This energy is used for everyday body functions such as heartbeat, digestion, breathing and movement. There are simple carbohydrates and complex carbohydrates. Simple carbohydrates have a chemical structure that is composed of either one or two sugars. Because they have a very simple chemical structure, they are quickly digested by the body. Examples of simple carbohydrates are table sugar, honey, agave nectar, white flour, juice, soda, cake, cookies, candy, chocolate, jam and sugared cereals. Simple carbohydrates are best to be limited because they don't sustain your body for a long period of time, they cause your blood sugar to spike and fall in a short period of time and you will require food again quickly. Complex carbohydrates are made up of more than two sugars. They are rich in fiber, vitamins and minerals and, because of their complex makeup, they take longer for the body to digest. They provide more sustainable energy than simple carbohydrates. Examples of complex carbohydrates are green, orange and yellow vegetables such as spinach, broccoli, yams, peppers, garlic, onions, squash, zucchini, eggplant, unflavored dairy products such as whole yogurt and milk, and legumes such as beans and peas.

Proteins are organic compounds that are made up of amino acids. Your body is made up almost completely of protein and all 20 amino acids must be present in order to maintain your bodily functions. Essential amino acids are those that are not manufactured in your body. Therefore you must get them from food sources. There are nine essential amino acids that you have to ingest via food to help your body continue to build, maintain and repair itself. Protein-containing foods are meat, fish, poultry, eggs, milk, cheese, yogurt, dark green leafy vegetables, tofu, soybeans, nuts and seeds.

Fat is made up of a glycerine molecule that has three fatty acids attached to it. Fat is a critical component for keeping your cells functioning properly, building tissue and regenerating cells; it insulates your body against shock, aids in the absorption of certain vitamins and minerals, keeps your body temperature stable and maintains healthy skin and hair. There are essential fatty acids that your body cannot manufacture and must come from food sources. These are Omega 3 and Omega 6 fatty acids. Some of the food sources that supply these essential fatty acids are fish, flaxseed, hemp oil, chia seeds, pumpkin seeds, sunflower seeds, leafy vegetables and walnuts.

Think of your body starting out each morning as an empty pegboard full of round holes. Each one of those holes needs to be filled with nutrients (round pegs) in order for your body to work efficiently. When you attempt to fill those holes with low nutrient or no nutrient foods (square pegs), they just don't get filled. But they still need to be, so of course your appetite will increase as you attempt to fill those holes. It would take more than 30 Snickers bars to get your full daily nutrients. That also equals about 8,500 calories, which is around four days' worth of food. Instead of all those candy bars to fill those holes, you could have 2 eggs for breakfast, plus 1 cup of oatmeal or yogurt and an apple. For lunch you could have a salmon filet, plus a spinach salad with dressing, avocado and tomato. For dinner you could have a six-ounce steak and a large sweet potato with butter. So, you can see here the difference between an empty calorie and a nutrient-filled calorie. Though it's true that a calorie is a calorie, not every calorie is nutritionally equal. You are going to get more bang for your buck if you go for whole foods. Eating empty calories won't be very satisfying if you are not filling those holes efficiently. Your body will feel fatigued and your mind, foggy. People who suffer from eating disorders often find that their brains just feel foggy due to lack of nutrients. They don't feel present and they have trouble being strong and grounded.

When you are ungrounded, you are not 'in your body'. You are disconnected with your physical needs, which also leads to binge eating. You are not getting the right calories, and your body will be begging you for nutrients. This will cause hunger and lead to erratic eating, which then becomes bingeing madly. This is part of the reason why you might have had the experience of being in a blackout where you were completely unaware of what you were doing until after the binge was over. This might have partly been your body's attempt to fill these nutritional holes.

This is not to say that empty calories should be avoided at all costs. That kind of rigidity and restriction can backfire. How many people do you know who have been on a no fat, no sugar, or no carbohydrate diet and then went on to binge on sweets after a few days? It's about paying attention to getting your nutrients in and then allowing a small percentage of your food to be just for fun. It's okay to even have a just for fun food every day. At the beginning of healing binge eating, that might have to wait awhile as fun foods can also be trigger foods, or foods that lead to a binge. As you feel stronger in your recovery, you can begin to incorporate foods that might have triggered a binge in the past, but no longer will.

At the beginning of recovery, when you are not quite eating complete whole healthy meals, it might be helpful to supplement with certain vitamins and minerals. A multivitamin with B complex vitamins can be helpful when trying to beat Binge Eating Disorder. B vitamins help your body to manufacture serotonin, a neurotransmitter that helps to regulate moods, sleep, and appetite. Vitamin B6 converts tryptophan into serotonin in your brain. Vitamin B12 also facilitates brain cell communication so that other neurotransmitters can work together to help relieve depression. In addition, this vitamin helps your body make use of chemicals such as dopamine and norepinephrine, which can help to promote a lighter mood.

Special Note to Vegetarians and Vegans

Ironically enough, many vegans and vegetarians suffer from Binge Eating Disorder. In my own experience of being a vegan for 15 years, I grudgingly learned that being a vegetarian was not the best diet for my body. It was very important for me to eat ethically and sustainably, but I was hungry, tired, foggy and dizzy a lot of the time. I accepted that state as normal. After attempting to cure my anemia for years with vegetarian iron supplements, I finally decided to just try to add a bit of animal protein in order to satisfy my doctor's pleas. I was completely shocked that after just a few days of eating small bits of eggs and some dairy that my intense food cravings had naturally died down. I was even more shocked when I began eating chicken and red meat and I was no longer dizzy. I had a much easier time with cognition and concentration after I began to eat meat again. It absolutely floored me. I decided to integrate meat into my diet again, which has improved my physical and my mental health immeasurably. However, having an omnivorous lifestyle isn't for everyone. If you are choosing a vegetarian or vegan lifestyle and you find yourself binge eating often, I would encourage you to consider experimenting with integrating wild fish, free-range fowl or grass-fed red meat into your diet for a few weeks. You might find that it makes a big difference in your cravings and compulsions. There are many who begin to add more animal protein into their diet and it simply cures their binge eating. One client even told me that she thought that eating ethical animal products sparingly was healthier for both her and the environment than when she was bingeing on prepackaged foods all the time. The waste that she created from empty chip bags, cake containers and cellophane wrappers was enormous.

Some vegans and vegetarians are binge eating because they are not eating the right foods to get the amount of protein and vitamins their bodies need. Some binge eaters use the excuse of a vegetarian or vegan lifestyle to put limits and restrictions on the amounts and kinds of foods that they eat. If you are eating a purely plant-based diet and you aren't diligent about getting proper nutrients you might find yourself hungry much of the time. When your body is hungry for nutrition, it will grab at whatever it can to help nourish it. This often happens without your permission. If you would prefer to maintain your vegetarian lifestyle, make sure that you're getting proper nutrition. Consider making an appointment with a vegetarian-friendly nutritionist. A vitamin won't trick your body into feeling satisfied, so you need to add whole food from plant sources to get the nutrients you need. By adding more fat into your diet in the form of nuts, seed, avocados, olive oil and coconut products, you will keep your appetite at bay so that binge eating won't be as driven by nutritional need. You should also look at adding complete proteins – those that contain all 20 amino acids such as amaranth, quinoa, buckwheat, soybeans and spirulina. If you are not vegan, consider adding butter and full fat dairy products.

Exercise: Proper On-hand Foods for You

Make a list of 10–15 whole foods: a combination of protein (i.e. meats, chicken, fish, eggs, dairy, nuts or tofu), carbohydrates (i.e. green vegetables, starchy vegetables, legumes, fruits and grains) and fats (oils, butter, nut butters) that you absolutely think of as low risk foods (foods you're not likely to binge on), and keep those in your house as staples. The following are my foods:

1. Apples, mangoes, berries (seasonal fruit)
2. Avocados
3. Eggs
4. Frozen grilled fully-cooked chicken breasts or strips
5. Raw nuts and seeds
6. Yams
7. Cans of tuna, salmon, and sardines
8. Bags of organic frozen vegetables (spinach, kale, broccoli, lima beans)
9. Cans of organic beans (black beans, kidney beans, garbanzo beans)
10. Pouches of tofu
11. Miso paste
12. Seaweed
13. Salsa

14. Butter

15. Amaranth/Quinoa

Your list might have different low risk high nutrition foods. But make these foods easy for you to grab and easy for you to prepare.

Step Eight – Plan on Eating Three Meals a Day

For many binge eaters, meals are erratic, inconsistent and riddled with guilt. Many try to go several hours without eating in order to compensate for eating too much and many eat way too much, way too often. Many skip breakfast and just opt for some coffee to get them going. This is especially true if they have a food hangover – that uncomfortable feeling one gets from a binge the night before.

One of the most important behavioral changes that you can make is to implement a normal eating pattern. That is three full meals a day and, if you need it, a snack or two.

Start by choosing a day that you will start. It doesn't matter if you binge the night before. No matter what, you are going to plan a regular day of eating *just this one day*. You might be scared. You might be terrified in fact if you've spent a long time skipping meals or restricting and bingeing, but just tell yourself that you're going to try this for one day. This doesn't have to be forever, this doesn't even have to be for a week, just once.

Set up a schedule for yourself as well as a meal plan. For example:

Meal:	Time:	Place:	Planned Food:
Breakfast	7am	Home	One cup of coffee with milk, medium-sized bowl of bran cereal with almond milk and a banana and 2 hard-boiled eggs.
Snack	10am	Work	One apple, and just one handful of almonds.

Lunch	1pm	Coffee shop near the office	One turkey sandwich on rye with lettuce, tomato and mustard, one orange, a small bag of chips, one bottle of spring water.
Snack	4pm	Office	One decaf latté with baby carrots and hummus.
Dinner	7pm	Home	One diced chicken breast sautéed with broccoli and mushrooms in olive oil and garlic, quinoa, one baked sweet potato with butter, asparagus.
Dessert	9pm	Home	One serving of ice cream.

Exercise One: Create a Meal Plan

Create your own food plan and vow to follow it for just one day. If you go to a restaurant, look online at the menu before you go in and plan what you will eat. Don't eat between your planned meals and snacks. You can find a meal planner in Appendix F or online.

Exercise Two: Figuring Out Why It's So Hard to Be a 'Normal' Eater – *Journal Opportunity*

1. I am/was afraid to implement a regular pattern of eating because:
2. When I tried this one-day experiment, I felt:
3. Things that were hard about it were:
4. Things that I liked about it were:
5. In order to integrate a regular pattern of eating into my daily life, I need to:

After you've done this for one whole day, choose two days in a row to implement the three-meal-a-day rule. Then, go for three days in a row, and so on. Eventually, you will find that you are eating three solid meals each day and not neglecting your hunger or eating when you are not hungry.

At the beginning, it's important to eat by the clock and eat according to your planned foods in order to stay accountable. If you find that you are unable to plan your actual meals for some reason, plan your meal times and limit yourself to only eating at those times.

When you get to the point that you are eating 3 full meals a day every day, you can let go of monitoring your food if you wish to, but continue to use your Alternative Action Log from Step Four if you have binged or if you are about to binge to continue understanding, monitoring and changing the disruptive behavior.

If you absolutely cannot commit to just one day of regular eating, start by committing to eating one healthy breakfast per week, then two healthy breakfasts per week, then three. Keep going until you are eating breakfast each morning. Next, conquer lunch. It is okay to do this slowly, but the start of a healthy breakfast each morning will set the tone for a healthy day.

Step Nine – Understanding Your Hunger

Part of knowing what you should eat is also beginning to understand hunger. Because so many disordered eaters lose track of the true sensation of hunger, eating can become a very confusing process. What you should eat, how much you should eat and when you should eat becomes stressful rather than intuitive. A large portion of the recovery process is relearning hunger and beginning to feed your body what it needs when it needs it.

You usually become aware that you are hungry when your stomach begins to growl. These hunger pangs are stomach contractions that send a signal to you that you are beginning to get hungry. The sense that you are finished eating is satiety, and that might manifest as the grumbling in your stomach subsiding, followed by the distension of your stomach and, if you continue to eat, an uncomfortable bloating of your intestines and belly.

CCK is the hormone that is released when food moves from the stomach to the intestines. It sends a signal to the hypothalamus that it's time to stop eating. Leptin is the hormone that is released by fat cells that decreases appetite when you've had enough food for your body.

So there are physical mechanisms and sensations set up to tell you how much to eat and the right foods to eat. Unfortunately, with binge eating, the psychological drive to eat becomes louder than the physical cues to stop.

In order to carry out the processes that keep your body alive, your body needs to be fed (given fuel). Thus, your body is in a continual state of hunger, which can be quickly relieved by eating. Having food present in your GI tract neutralizes the feeling of hunger, which helps you to feel calm both physically and emotionally. Once your body metabolizes this food and utilizes it to carry out the functions that it needs to survive, you feel hungry again and it's time to eat.

Simple. But not really, right?

If hunger were such a basic biological process, then no one with access to food would ever starve or overeat, right? Well clearly that's not the case. Somehow, along the way, when food became plentiful and a doctrine of thin became dictatorially pervasive, our minds and bodies began to disagree on what we should eat and how much we should eat.

Most disordered eaters have absolutely no idea when they're hungry or when they've had enough. Those who do not suffer from disordered eating know when they are hungry and feed themselves what their bodies need. This is not the case with a typical disordered eater. Chronic dieters learn how to deny their hunger. Some people equate feeling hungry with being good and virtuous. Binge eaters eat until they are uncomfortably full, completely surpassing the feeling of being satisfied.

Many people are never in touch with their own cues for hunger and satiety. Often, well-meaning parents force their children to eat because they fear that their kids aren't getting enough food. This then causes kids not to trust their own bodily signals. As they grow up, they believe that they should clean their plates without checking with their body as to whether or not they need more. Many people eat until they are unable to eat any more.

We have more access to food and we have more rules about what our bodies are supposed to look like. Food is everywhere, it's advertised all over the place, but so are promises of an ultra thin body if you follow *this one diet* – **the very last diet you will ever need**. It's not uncommon to be watching TV when a commercial for an unending pasta bowl comes on followed by an advertisement for a prepackaged food diet program. Wait. What? It's kind of insane. It's like the media wants us to have eating disorders because it's the only way all sides win. EAT! EAT! EAT! STARVE! STARVE! STARVE! EAT! STARVE! EAT! STARVE! EAT! STARVE!

It's incredibly confusing, and messes with our ability to understand what we need or don't need physically.

No wonder our cues for hunger and satiety are so out of whack. If you have been on or off a diet, you've gotten the message somewhere, probably at some young age, that you should be thin and so you begin to deny your hunger. Then, of course, you binge because humans are biologically predisposed to overeat after times of restriction to keep our physiological processes going. This is a survival mechanism – just in case you are restricted food again, you must binge to stay alive. Think prehistoric man and the feast or famine phenomena. But after your summer of bingeing on berries and bears, instead of settling into your cave for a long winter of sleep, sex, and little food, you barricade yourself into your bedroom full of guilt, full of shame, full of anxiety; and you either start some kind of new diet to gain control or you eat compulsively to stuff the feelings of stress and anxiety. Cravings become difficult to distinguish from real physiological hunger and so you begin to deny real hunger, and because you're not giving in to your 'cravings', you confuse the feeling of deep hunger with virtuosity, self-control and willpower.

When you don't eat enough, your body begins to shut down. You become tired. Your body tries to conserve what it has to carry out basic functions such as respiration. When you go long periods of time without eating, your organs shut down and you die. This is what happens with anorexia and unintentional starvation.

When you eat more than your body needs, you are overloaded with energy in the form of calories and your body has to work extra hard to process that food. This is part of why people often feel sluggish and tired the day after a binge.

Exercise One: Do You Understand When You are Hungry and When You are Full?

1. When you *think* that you are hungry, ask yourself how you know that you're hungry before you eat anything. Sometimes people think they're physically hungry, but they're actually bored, procrastinating, tired, anxious, lonely, angry, stressed, sad, happy or thirsty.
2. Check in with your physical cues for hunger. These signs might be your stomach growling, pain in your abdomen, a feeling of emptiness, a lack of energy, fogginess, lack of concentration, a headache or dizziness. Your body will let you know when it is ready for more food.
3. If you are not having any physical cues of hunger, see if you can wait 10–15 minutes and do something else. Set a timer and walk around the block. If you are obsessing on food, think about what it is that you actually need. Sometimes it's easier to just eat than to deal with the real issue at hand. Food is always there if you need it, but push yourself a little bit to tend to your other needs. Eating can be a way of neglecting your other needs.
4. Don't neglect your body if you are hungry. Feed yourself.

Exercise Two: Learning Hunger and Satiety Scale

The hunger and satiety scale helps you to relearn your hunger. Keep it in your wallet and check in with yourself often during the day to see where your hunger lies in the scale:

Hunger & Satiety Scale

0 – Beyond Hunger

At this point, you have denied your hunger for so long that you don't even have any symptoms of hunger. Your body is in starvation mode. Your metabolism is slowing down. You probably feel low energy, tired and empty.

1 – Ravenous

You feel like you're starving. Your body is just looking for nutrients before it shuts down and you begin running on adrenaline. This is the place where many people binge. Your body needs food now and will eat as much as it possibly can to get the nutrients it needs to run without you having the power to intervene.

2 – Very Hungry

You are thinking about food a great deal now, unable to focus on work or conversations.

3 – Hungry

You notice that your stomach might be beginning to growl, you begin to lose your focus a bit, and you are becoming distracted easily.

4 – Almost Hungry

This is when your first thoughts of food begin, or, if while you are eating, you stop too soon, still feeling as though you need more food.

5 – Neutral

At this point, you don't feel hungry, nor do you feel full. You are not fixated or even thinking about food. You are able to be productive, and focus on work or conversation.

6 – Satisfied

You have eaten enough to feel content. You have fed yourself what your body needs. You are no longer hungry, yet you are not feeling too full. You are able to stop eating at this moment if you want.

7 – Slightly Full

You are a little more than satisfied, you are aware of the feeling of food in your stomach, possibly feeling as though you've had a few bites too many.

8 – Very Full

You are feeling your belly pushing out, you feel like you've had too much.

9 – Uncomfortably Full

Your body feels uncomfortable. You just want to go to sleep at this point. You might be feeling depressed or regretful.

10 – Completely Stuffed

At this point, you feel like you might throw up. You have eaten so much that you are in pain. Your belly hurts and you can't focus on anything else. You might just want to go to bed.

When using the hunger and satiety scale, you should try not to let yourself get lower than a 3 or higher than a 7. Meals and snacks should be slow and mindful to allow you to understand what your body needs.

I understand that many of you will look at this hunger and satiety scale and be more confused about your hunger than ever. I can't tell you how many patients have come in and looked at me with confusion when I've shown them this chart, and said to me, "But I don't even understand what it means to be hungry or to be full. I have no idea what it feels like."

So, for many of you, it's time to learn.

First off, you might notice that you believe you are hungry when your appetite is stimulated. It could be triggered by outside stimulus, such as smelling a certain food, seeing someone eat something, or watching a commercial for a certain food on television. And, as I have been saying throughout the book, hunger can also be your automatic response to anxiety, depression, fear, happiness or other feelings. Hunger and therefore eating might be your unconscious coping mechanism to temporarily block out these feelings. You believe that you are hungry, but you're really sad or anxious and your unconscious mind leads you toward food to make the sadness disappear.

Trixie, a 34-year-old patient of mine, suffered intensely from clinical depression. The more depressed she became, the more weight she gained. She told me one day that food was the only thing that made her happy. I asked her if it made her happy or if it just momentarily blocked out her sadness. She acquiesced that it's probably what that was. She was so afraid to deal with her depression, that she allowed the food to take over, causing her great medical issues, and a body that held close to 400 pounds. Her depression caused her weight, and her weight caused her depression. She often believed that she would be happy if she lost weight, and worked vehemently on trying to lose that weight. But until she focused on her depression and what was really going on with herself emotionally, her weight remained a problem to her.

In order to begin to understand your hunger, you need to begin to notice what happens both in your body and what happens for you emotionally. Some people find that any feelings of hunger create extreme uneasiness for them. Jennifer, another patient of mine, had a great deal of anxiety about not getting enough to eat. She would hoard food and any light pang of hunger would send her into an intense anxiety state. As a child, after her father left, her mother had very little money to feed the family. They survived day to day, not always knowing whether or not they would have food or shelter. As an adult, although Jennifer was quite well off, her survival instincts still told her that food was not plentiful and that if she were hungry, she would surely die of starvation. Intellectually, she knew that it was impossible; but her unconscious mind, the little girl inside of her, had a very different reality. Because of this, she was vigilant about never allowing herself to become hungry. If she was in a place where she knew she wouldn't be able to eat for a period of time, she became incredibly anxious and began to avoid meetings at work or business trips. Her fear began to limit her significantly. If she knew that she had to be in a meeting or take a trip in a car, she would binge before she left and take extra food with her, even for an hour-long meeting. As she began to become more comfortable with allowing herself to wait to eat until she was hungry, she began to understand that light hunger would not kill her. She actually did not know what it meant to be hungry. As a child, her mom would often tell her that they had no money for food, and that they would certainly starve. As an adult, understanding that starvation was not a real threat for her was very helpful.

Exercise Three: Learning What Real Hunger Feels Like in Your Body – *Journal Opportunity*
Warning: Do not do this exercise without first consulting with your physician

In preparation for this exercise, set aside a day when you don't have to go to work or have social plans. Find someone who will join you for the day to do things between journal sessions like watch movies or chat. Plan three non-binge meals that are each made up of protein, fat and carbohydrates. When you wake up in the morning, have a moderate breakfast. It is important that you do this on a day where you have not binged the night before. Try to include protein, fat, fiber, carbohydrates and vitamins in this breakfast. Something like 2 eggs scrambled with a bit of cheese, one piece of fruit and one or two slices of whole grain toast with butter. After your meal, wait. At two hours, begin to check in with your body and notice if you have any signs of hunger. These signs might be your stomach growling, pain in your stomach, a feeling of emptiness, a lack of energy, fogginess, lack of concentration, headache, dizziness, obsessing about food, or other feelings.

At the two-hour mark, fill in the following chart:

Hunger Symptom	Do you have this? (yes/no)	What number on the hunger/satiety scale?
Stomach Growling		
Stomach Pains		
Hollow Feelings		
Lack of Energy		

Fogginess
Lack of Concentration
Headache
Dizziness
Obsessing about Food
Other Feelings

Notice what you are feeling emotionally. In your journal, note what feelings are coming up for you. Are you feeling anxious about food? Are you feeling angry? Sad? What are you thinking about?

Now, wait another hour. When it's been three hours since you've eaten, begin to check your symptoms and mark them down:

Hunger Symptom	Do you have this? (yes/no)	What number on the hunger/satiety scale?
Stomach Pains		
Hollow Feelings		
Lack of Energy		
Fogginess		
Lack of Concentration		
Headache		
Dizziness		
Obsessing about Food		
Other Feelings		

Notice what you are feeling emotionally. What feelings are coming up for you? Are you feeling anxious about food? Are you feeling angry? Sad? What are you thinking about? Another feeling that might be coming up for you around hunger is elation. For some people, the feeling of being empty is desirable. They might feel more in control, safer and, in some cases, morally superior.

Now, wait another hour. When it's been four hours since you've eaten, begin to check your symptoms and mark them down.

Hunger Symptom	Do you have this? (yes/no)	What number on the hunger/satiety scale?
Stomach Pains		
Hollow Feelings		
Lack of Energy		
Fogginess		
Lack of Concentration		
Headache		
Dizziness		
Obsessing about Food		
Other Feelings		

Notice what you are feeling emotionally. What feelings are coming up for you? Are you feeling anxious about food? Are you feeling angry? Sad? What are you thinking about?

Now, wait another hour. When it's been five hours since you've eaten, begin to check your symptoms and mark them down.

Hunger Symptom	Do you have this? (yes/no)	What number on the hunger/satiety scale?
Stomach Pains		
Hollow Feelings		
Lack of Energy		
Fogginess		
Lack of Concentration		
Headache		
Dizziness		
Obsessing about Food		
Other Feelings		

Notice what you are feeling emotionally. What feelings are coming up for you? Are you feeling anxious about food? Are you feeling angry? Sad? What are you thinking about?

At the six-hour mark, you should definitely be quite hungry. Allow yourself to check in one last time. At this point you should definitely understand what hunger feels like emotionally and physically. Check in again and mark off what you are feeling physically and emotionally.

Hunger Symptom	Do you have this? (yes/no)	What number on the hunger/satiety scale?
Stomach Pains		
Hollow Feelings		
Lack of Energy		
Fogginess		
Lack of Concentration		
Headache		
Dizziness		
Obsessing about Food		
Other Feelings		

Notice what you are feeling emotionally. What feelings are coming up for you? Are you feeling anxious about food? Are you feeling angry? Sad? What are you thinking about?

As you continue on your journey, continue to notice what physical and emotional cues of hunger you are having. You will begin to understand more about what and when to eat.

At this point, allow yourself to eat a full non-binge meal. Try to eat slowly and to notice as you go from being hungry to being satisfied. Because you are so hungry and because you might have lots of emotions coming up for you from this exercise, you might find that you have the instinct to eat very quickly to make the hunger and the feelings disappear. Slow yourself down and notice what truly satisfying your hunger feels like. Try to stop when you are at a 6, when you are satisfied, but not full. As you continue on your journey, each meal should start at a 3 and end by a 6 or 7.

You should not end your meals by saying, "I'm so full." You should feel sated and nourished.

Exercise Four: Understanding the Cues that Cause You to Eat – *Journal Opportunity*

The next time you eat anything, sit down afterwards and answer these questions:

1. Were you physically hungry?
2. If you were physically hungry, how did you know that? What were the bodily cues that told you to eat?
3. Were you psychologically hungry?
4. If you were psychologically hungry, what were you hungry for? What did you need emotionally? Were you bored, tired, angry, lonely? What else could have fed you?
5. Were you eating as a conditioned response? For example, popcorn at a movie, or snack after work?
6. If so, is there a way that you could notice this in the future?

Exercise Five: The Mindful Meal

A planned mindful meal is an intentional space that you create to understand more about your feelings when you are eating, as well as to help you tune in to your hunger, satiety and your digestion. The more mindful meals that you do, the more you will begin to understand the difference between real physical hunger and fake hunger that is triggered by an external force.

Preparation:
1. Set aside a time when you can be alone and without distraction.

2. Turn off your television, turn off your computer, and turn off your iPhone.

3. If you need a bit of stimulation, you can listen to light meditative music or some classical music.

4. Make sure that the lights are all on.

5. Slowly and with care, prepare a meal for yourself. Use all of your senses, notice what it's like to prepare your food. Take time to notice the colors and smells of your food. Feel the tactile sensation of cutting your vegetables and meat. Hear the sizzling of food cooking, but allow yourself to wait to taste.

6. Don't eat any food or snack during the preparation. You will not eat until you are sitting at the table.

7. Create a welcoming table setting for yourself. Use your favorite dishes, and perhaps light some candles, use your favorite tablecloth. Set some flowers and make it beautiful for yourself.

The Meal:

1. As you sit down, before you begin to eat, check in with your body and assess where you are on the hunger and satiety scale.

2. Before you start to eat, look down at your food and see what is on your plate.

3. Take a breath, you might want to send a word of gratitude, or just give yourself a positive affirmation. Make an intention for the meal. It might be, "I choose to eat slowly" or "I choose to stop eating when I am satisfied whether or not there is still food on my plate" or "I choose to allow myself to eat free of guilt or shame." Think about what is important to you.

4. Decide what you want to eat first.

5. Put that first forkful of food into your mouth and really taste it.

6. Taste and thoroughly chew each bite and put your fork down after every two bites.

7. Notice your thoughts and feelings as you eat without engaging with them, just noticing what happens when you allow yourself to really *be* with your food.

8. When you are halfway done with the content of your meal, stop, put your fork down, take a few deep breaths and notice where you are on the hunger and satiety scale.

9. If you are at 3, 4, or 5, allow yourself to eat more, and then stop when you are halfway done with the contents of what is on your plate and assess again. Continue to do this until you are at a 6.

10. When you are at a 6 or higher, put your fork down and put your food away for later.

Give yourself permission to get up from the table and do something else.

Notice what you are feeling. Are you anxious? Do you want to eat more? Are you able to go about your business or are you obsessing about food?

If so, what would you be thinking about if you weren't thinking about food?

Your body is no longer hungry, so you don't need food. You need something else, but what might that be? Sit with that feeling of wanting and allow yourself to go deeper.

Call your support person and let them know that you want to eat, but you know you are not hungry. Ask them if they are open to exploring what you might need right then.

If you are unable to do that, sit down and write in a journal about what you are experiencing. Allow that feeling of anxiety and the obsession with the food to pass right through you.

If you never get to a 6 while eating, you might be underestimating how much food you need. You might want to experiment with putting more food on your plate.

Doing this exercise at least once per week can really help you to tune in to both your emotional needs and your physical needs. It will help you to be more conscious about binge eating and emotional eating vs. eating for nourishment and sustenance. As you continue on your journey, you will find a consciousness that did not previously exist bringing your unconscious behaviors out into the open so that you are more in control of what you choose to do. As you slow down, your body will inform you of what you need.

Exercise Six: Mindfulness Journey – *Meditation Time*

Close your eyes and check in with your body. Notice the position that you're in. Notice your feet on the floor, the bend of your knees in the chair that you're in, the way your head feels... really let yourself feel what it's like to be in your body. Stretch if your body wants to stretch, bend if your body wants to bend, roll your wrists, your neck, your ankles, whatever you need.

Next, do a body scan. Start by noticing the bottoms of your feet and slowly make your way to the top of your head, feeling into each part of your body and noticing what's happening. Do you notice itches? Cricks? Muscle tightness? Aches? Soreness? Tingles? Hunger? Thirst? Emptiness? Fullness? Cramps? See what physical feeling is screaming out for your attention, and just be with that feeling for a few moments, without judging it, without trying to change it. Name it. For instance, your nose is itching, breathe into it and say, "Itchy nose." If your shoulders are tight breathe into them and state, "Tight shoulders," and just breathe for a few moments into whatever part wants your attention.

Then ask your body, "What do you need?" Your body might say, "More water," or "More kindness," or "More vegetables," or "More fresh air..." It might tell you that it needs fat or it might need carbohydrates or it might need protein. Be still. Sit, listen and just hear what your body is telling you. When you are in your body, you know exactly what you need. When you are in your body, you are more likely to nurture and care for it rather than treat it poorly with bingeing, restricting, too much exercise, too little exercise.

Deciphering Physical Hunger from Other Physical Symptoms

As you begin to understand your hunger, you might find that things you used to think were hunger were actually other physical symptoms that you used to associate with hunger. For instance, you might believe that you are hungry when you are actually dehydrated. You might want to drink a glass of water to see if you are actually thirsty. Another feeling people often confuse with hunger is fatigue. You might be both physically and emotionally tired. You might need a nap rather than to eat. These are things to ponder.

Keeping Safe Non-Binge Foods Around

Because it's important to make sure that you don't let yourself get too hungry, keeping accessible, filling, non-binge foods close at hand is vital. One patient of mine bought an extra large purse that she always kept some hard-boiled eggs and apples in. She knew that those were foods that would satisfy her, but that she wouldn't have to risk bingeing on. There are many foods that are touted as great snack foods, yet for many people they are binge foods. You have to be honest with yourself about what you binge on and what you don't. Many people find that certain 'healthy snack foods', such as pretzels, nuts, yogurt drops, puffs, can trigger a binge.

Are there some healthy foods that you are prone to binge on? If so, these should not be easily accessible to you while you are recovering from binge eating.

Step Ten – Overpowering Your Urge to Binge

Imagine that your urge to binge is a parasite called the binge monster that lives on you. The binge monster is fed every time you give in to your urge to binge. Because this urge is a parasite, it relies on you to feed it, nurture it and keep it alive. You keep it alive by bingeing. Each time you binge, you make it stronger. Every time you have the urge to binge, it's the binge monster demanding its fix. When you don't feed it, you feel so anxious and so distressed. However, this is not you. This is the binge monster beginning to feel distressed. It knows that if you don't binge, it starves. The more you starve it the weaker it gets. It will try really hard to get you to feed it. It is in survival mode. It wants to live. The stronger you become, the more you refuse to feed it, the weaker it becomes. You are stronger than your urge to binge. It pretends to be a big scary monster, but it is really a weak little child, begging for attention. Eventually, if you continue to deny that urge, the binge monster will become weaker and weaker. You will become stronger and stronger and eventually the parasite will die. Every time you refuse to give in to your binge monster, you strengthen yourself. You strengthen your freedom of choice and your own decision-making skills.

Exercise One: Personifying Your Bingeing – *Journal Opportunity*

The point of this exercise is to help you to gain some power over your binge eating. By externalizing your binge eating and recognizing that it is not an inseparable part of yourself, you are able to detach yourself from the disorder. Some people think that they are a walking eating disorder, but you are not. You are a whole, solid human being with an issue that needs attention and a behavior that you'd like to extinguish. You are not hopeless. I have seen so many people heal from this disorder and I know that you can too.

Answer the following questions in your journal:

1. What is the name of your binge monster? Think about the parasite that comes and has you bingeing before you even believe that you have a choice; what will you call this entity?
2. What does it look like? Describe it in words.
3. How long has it been living on you/in you?
4. When did she or he first attach himself/herself onto you? How old were you? What were the circumstances surrounding it?
5. Draw a picture of your binge monster.
6. Write a letter to your binge monster letting it know how you feel about it. Ask it what its purpose is, and why it has chosen to come to you.
7. Write a letter to yourself from your binge monster, explaining why he or she is there, and whatever else he or she wants you to know.
8. Write a letter back to your binge monster explaining why you don't need him or her, and what coping mechanisms you have to deal with life other than him or her. Ask him or her to gently let go of you.

Meditation Time

Close your eyes and visualize yourself standing in front of your binge monster. If your binge monster puffs out his chest, you puff your chest out more. If your binge monster makes a big scary face or gnashes his teeth, you make a scarier face and roar at him. See yourself getting bigger while your binge monster shrinks. Tell him that you refuse to support him and keep him alive any longer. The point of this exercise is to help remind your consciousness that you have a choice when you are thinking of bingeing. You will remember that you can fight this monster because you are strong too. Sometimes just remembering that you are bigger than the urge to binge can shift your consciousness enough to help you make the decision not to binge when the option presents itself.

Exercise Two: Delaying and Interrupting a Binge

Now that you've thrown away your bathroom scale, it's time to replace it with a new piece of equipment, the kitchen timer. This is your first defense against a binge. The next time you get the urge to binge or to eat one of your trigger foods, set the timer for 20 minutes and tell yourself that if after 20 minutes you still want to binge or to eat your trigger food, you still can. You can do this even if you've already started a binge. You are allowed to interrupt a binge. It doesn't have to be all or nothing. What you're aiming for here is moderation. Stopping in the middle of a binge is great progress. It shows that you are getting away from the binge mentality, which is all about all or nothing thinking.

During the 20 minutes that the timer is set, try to think about why you've decided to binge and what you are feeling. If you'd prefer not to think, you can also go to your Do Something Different List and do one of those activities for the 20 minutes. Remember, you are not trying to stop yourself from bingeing; you are just attempting to bring some mindfulness to the situation. Once you interrupt the compulsion, the binge is no longer in charge; you now have the ability to decide whether or not this is what you really want rather than letting the impulse to binge do it for you. Although it feels like the binge is in charge, you are stronger than your impulse to binge.

When the 20 minutes is over, see if you still want to binge. If so, try to let yourself do it consciously. It's amazing how different an experience it will be when you let yourself be present for the binge. All of a sudden, you have some say over what happens.

You have the ability to decide what you eat and how much you eat. You can choose whether or not this is a big out of control binge, a contained snack, or something completely different.

Step Eleven – Increasing Your Tolerance for Uncomfortable Feelings

As you begin to differentiate between physical hunger and emotional hunger, you might begin to feel uncomfortable. You've spent so many years using food and dieting to stuff down your feelings; and without these obsessions, they all rise to the surface. Choosing not to do anything to make those feelings go away and learning how to sit with those feelings is challenging. Part of the reason we binge eat is to avoid feeling what is really going on. If you can just acknowledge what you feel and say it out loud, then just take five minutes to sit with it without doing anything about it; you will find that it becomes easier to be with your feelings. All you have to do is acknowledge your feeling, name it, and then just be with it for a bit. Let yourself feel it.

Remember that "fat" is not a feeling. It's a descriptor and a judgment. If you are "feeling fat" you are judging yourself and your body. What is the feeling underneath that judgment? Is it pain? Sadness? Anxiety?

Look through the feelings list below and see what feelings you might be able to identify with:

Pleasant Feelings
Happy
Excited
Alive
Enthusiastic
Jubilant
Interested
Calm
Peaceful
Safe

Blessed
Joyous
Thankful
Cheerful
Free
Playful
Lucky
Thrilled
Independent
Accepting
Compassionate
Kind
Confident
In love
Loved
Loving
Maternal
Brave
Strong
Smart
Bold
Curious

Challenging Feelings
Lonely
Sad
Angry
Anxious
Furious
Hostile
Confused
Hurt
Embarrassed
Frustrated

Useless
Hopeless
Longing
Desire
Guilt
Shame
Misunderstood
Tired
Exhausted
Disgusted
Appalled
Shocked
Betrayed
Inferior
Powerless
Manipulated
Vulnerable
Hesitant
Mistrustful
Victimized
Enraged
Paralyzed
Nothing
Desperate
Grieving
Threatened
Scared
Unsafe
Wary
Bored
Procrastinating
Worried

This is not about making your feelings go away, it's about becoming comfortable with them, even if they are so uncomfortable that you want to hide. If you can be okay with the fact that you are having these feelings, and sit with the discomfort, then you don't need to use food to comfort or temporarily distract yourself from them.

When I first began seeing Kensey, she had no idea of what she was feeling. She had been using food to numb out since she was a teenager. When I asked her what she was feeling, she would look at me for a moment and say, "I feel fine." Fine isn't a feeling.

"I feel fat," she would then tell me. Fat isn't a feeling either.

A feeling is an experience of an emotional state. We tend to categorize feelings in terms of good and bad; happiness is good, but anger or sadness is bad. As children, for many of us, our parents would feel angry or frustrated when we cried or became angry. Although anger and sadness are normal, everyday feelings, we became conditioned to believe that they were not okay. As human beings, we have come equipped with millions of feelings and states of being, yet we believe it's only okay to feel one way. Fine. Not happy, not sad. Just nothing. Fine.

Feelings aren't wrong or bad. Feelings just are. Sadness isn't bad, but it is hard to feel, and when we feel sadness or anger, we want to do things like cry, or writhe on the floor or the bed, kicking and screaming. But we are not children; we are adults and feeling that way is judged as bad or wrong. A binge eater will take that feeling and stuff it down with food in order not to feel it. All feelings are worthy of being felt. They give you a message about what you need. Letting yourself experience your feelings allows you to take action and choose to give yourself what you need, or it allows feelings to pass through. There are certain situations such as clinical depression or anxiety disorders when moods can take over emotions. In cases like this, psychotherapy and psychopharmacological interventions can be extremely helpful in healing these psychological disorders. What can be so challenging is that when you stop your binge eating behaviors, other, more challenging feelings, begin to arise. This is where your work really begins. As you begin to feel less afraid of your feelings, you will find that you don't need food to stuff them down. This is also when many people want to quit, when all the feelings that they had been suppressing begin to arise. Just know that this is a natural part of recovery and things will shift as you become stronger and more confident and allow yourself to be who you really are.

Exercise: Feeling the Feelings – *Meditation Time*

- Look over the feelings list.
- Assess what you might be feeling.
- Notice where in your body you feel it.
- Once you identify the feeling and where you are holding it, just sit with it, say it out loud and breathe into that part of your body.
- You might notice that one of your feelings is the urge to binge. You might even feel obsessed.
- Just because you want to binge so badly does not mean that you don't have the capacity to sit with it.
- You might feel the urge to binge in your jaw.
- Just put your hands on your jaw and say or think the word "Urge" or "Obsession."
- Breathe into it and let it move through you.

Your feelings can be bearable. When you sit with your feelings without judgment, without fear, without trying to make them go away, you increase your capacity to sit with them and eventually they move. Often, the need to push a feeling away can be more stressful and challenging than the feeling itself.

When you are feeling sad, the last thing that you need is judgment and self-flagellation about your feelings. This just intensifies your challenging feelings. Allowing yourself to acknowledge them, accept them and be with them will help them move through you. For example, you might notice that you feel anxiety in your belly. Sit down, put your hand on your belly and just repeat the word "Anxiety" as you hold your belly. Just begin to breathe into that part of your body and let it move through you. Let yourself understand that you can sit with these feelings. If you find it impossible to sit with these feelings, please do talk to a professional who can help you to deal with them more efficiently.

Right now, it's just important to learn how to sit with these feelings in order to increase your capacity to be with uncomfortable feelings. In Step Nineteen, we will discuss more of what to do with these feelings.

Step Twelve – Balancing Self-Acceptance with the Need to Change

The most challenging task that I have with my patients is self-acceptance.

I worked with Alex, a 29-year-old brilliant woman who insisted that it was absolutely wrong for her to accept herself when she had 30 extra pounds on her. Alex felt that self-acceptance was not okay when it was her belief that she had so much weight to lose.

"Why is that?" I asked her.

"I don't deserve to accept myself at this weight. I'm disgusting, and if I do accept myself then I will become even more fat, lazy, and disgusting."

"So," I asked, "what happens when you hate yourself?"

"It makes me work harder."

"And how long have you been binge eating?"

"Since I was 8 or 9, maybe even before that... I don't know, maybe always."

"And does hating and berating yourself help you to refrain from bingeing?"

"No. But I don't see how accepting myself will. I motivate myself by telling myself that I'm fat, lazy and disgusting. That's how I get myself to do what I need to do."

The irony here is that in order to change, you have to accept what is. Alex's self-hatred was a self-perpetuating issue. She disliked herself, felt she deserved to stay in an emotionally abusive relationship, felt that she was less-than and had no voice in her relationship, felt alone and isolated, so she binged, the binges caused her to feel anger, shame and self-hatred, and so she binged again. Her boyfriend was constantly chastising her and telling her that she was too fat and lazy. She believed him because she felt the same way; she believed that she was worthless because of her weight, and if she could change that, everything would be fine. She never looked at her relationship, just at her eating behavior. She believed that her relationship would get better when she lost weight. This cycle is vicious and pervasive. It's impossible to change anything without accepting the reality of the situation. The reality is, "I have an issue with binge eating." Can you accept that? That is the only thing that you have to accept. You accept it without judgment; it isn't good and it isn't bad. It just is. Are you able to accept that you would like to change this behavior? Okay. That's all you need to know for the moment. You have a problem with binge eating. The first step in any recovery program is acceptance. Allow yourself to say it out loud, "I have a problem with binge eating and I accept that. This doesn't make me a bad person; this just makes me a person with a binge eating issue. I also accept that I want to change this behavior pattern." You will find that it is easier on your constitution to sit in acceptance than in judgment.

Alex had quite a traumatic childhood. Her mother and stepfather were horribly abusive toward her. Alex grew up constantly being given the message that there was something wrong with her. She was to cook, clean, and give in to her stepfather sexually. She was a modern day Cinderella – neglected, forced to do housework, beaten and molested. Her mother only paid attention to her when she was yelling at her to get things done. Her stepfather only paid attention to her when he was sexually abusing her. Because of this neglect, Alex had to grab food where and when she could. She would sneak eat when her mother was away or sleeping. Because she was only able to receive any kind of nourishment by stealing food and hoarding it, she learned how to nourish herself emotionally in that way. Because she was forced to do so much hard labor and was paid attention to when she was being commanded and abused, she believed that in order to get something done she had to abuse herself. She then became a victim to herself. She refused to accept who she was and where she was in the moment. Alex is an extreme case of refusing to accept oneself. Alex's severe trauma was stored in her body. In many cases of extreme abuse, the trauma lasts a lifetime. All the incidents of touching, hitting, harming are still deeply felt. It was impossible for Alex to accept her body because it had been so violated. In fact, she often was not even in her body. Bingeing was a way for her to dissociate – or to leave her body. Accepting her body would mean accepting the abuse and the shame that she felt with it. Alex worked with me for years and as she allowed herself to be with her story, she began to accept herself as a whole and complete human being. She was not someone who was flawed; she was someone who was victimized by sick people. As she realized that, she began to heal. She became empowered in her own body and began to accept who she was as a person underneath the abuse. She was not her abuse nor was she her abuser. As she healed and grew stronger, she found that she didn't have to change, that she was perfect the way she was. She didn't have to leave her body or change her body to be a better person. She was totally perfect already. Upon realizing that, she left her emotionally abusive relationship. Ironically, she began to let go of her binge eating at this point. She did drop the weight that she wanted to, almost without realizing it. She had found more peace within and stopped relying on food to hide from her SELF. She accepted her traumatic history, and began to use it as a vehicle for transformation and growth.

Another patient, Chloe, was a very high functioning overachiever who had two graduate degrees from Ivy League schools. Though she came from a loving and supportive family, she motivated herself by constantly comparing herself to others and believing that she didn't measure up so she had to compete. This happened a hundredfold when it came to her body. She was always comparing her body to other women's bodies. She would then be convinced that she wasn't good enough, berate herself, diet, binge, hate herself, diet, binge, hate herself, diet, binge, hate herself…

Self-acceptance was not an easy journey for her, but she came to realize that she had a path that was uniquely her own, that she could not be like others because she was not others – she was Chloe. She stopped striving to be better than other people, acknowledging that there was no 'better' or 'worse' when it came to people, there was just different. She committed to being one great Chloe and accepted herself completely. Self-acceptance gave her the ability to be okay with who she was without comparing herself to others which then allowed her to stop dieting, which then allowed her to stop bingeing.

Self-acceptance is not easy when you are used to berating yourself. It does not mean becoming complacent; it means loving who you are no matter where you're at. Self-acceptance means having an understanding that you might be in this place right now, but you have the ability to evolve and move through this space. It's not about accepting that things will never change, but about saying, "Okay, I'm here today, I might not be tomorrow. Tomorrow is another day. There is always an opportunity for growth."

Exercise One: Self-Acceptance – *Journal Opportunity*
Complete the following sentences:

I am afraid of accepting myself as I am because:
If I were to accept my body shape, I might feel:
If I were to accept my eating issues, I might feel:
The bad thing about accepting my eating issues is:
The bad thing about accepting my body shape is:
A positive thing that might happen if I accept my eating issues is:
A good thing that might happen if I accept my body shape is:

Exercise Two: Releasing Judgment

Many people who are very self-critical also tend to be outwardly critical and judgmental to the people around them. Take one day and vow to try to notice your judgments on people. They might be as simple as, "That person shouldn't be wearing those pants," or as complex as, "My friend Joanna is a very bad mother."

Choose one day and every time you notice a judgment, take note of how it feels in your body. Try to replace the judgment with a kind or compassionate statement about that person, for example, "I might not like those pants, but I don't have to wear them, and she certainly has kind eyes. Wearing the right pants is probably not one of her priorities, and I am respectful of that," or "Joanna is a very different kind of parent than I am, but her son Dimitri seems well-adjusted; I must respect that everyone has their own parenting styles."

Notice the difference you feel in your body. Some people report feeling lighter and not having as much holding them down when they do this exercise. Many people report feeling more space for compassion for themselves and for others without the judgments to hold them down.

Choose another day, and for every person you come in contact with, allow yourself to try and see the good in each person. Smile and think of one kind thing to say about each person in your mind. You can even say these things out loud if you like. The important thing is to feel kindness and compassion in your body rather than judgment and criticism.

Choose another day. This is for drivers. Allow yourself to drive very considerately, allowing people to pass you, allowing people to go ahead of you in a four-way stop sign intersection, allowing space for people who are trying to get out of a parking spot or driveway. How does that feel in your body? We hold so much stress driving, trying to get ahead of people. It's always relaxing to try and let go of that, not to mention safer.

Exercise Three: Finding Positive Qualities –
Journal Opportunity

Make a list of things that you like about yourself and what you feel your positive qualities are:

Make a list of things that you don't like about yourself and what you feel your negative qualities are:

Do your bad qualities make you a bad person? Why or Why Not?

Do your bad qualities take away from your good qualities? Why or Why Not?

Can you accept that you have both bad and good qualities? Why or Why Not?

Exercise Four: The Mirror Exercise

Stand in front of a mirror and gaze into your eyes; let your gaze fall onto your face. Is there something there that you like? Can you look deep inside your eyes and see the person who is truly there, beyond just the physical appearance? Can you accept that person? Can you send that person loving compassion?

Some thoughts to send yourself in the mirror:

- I know that this is a struggle, but you are trying hard and doing the best you can. I will be here for you.
- You deserve love and respect. I will do my best to love and respect you.
- I am sorry for the pain I've caused you; I am learning to be kinder to you now.
- Binge eating is hard to conquer, but I am here for you.
- Just because you have this issue doesn't make you a bad person. You have been doing the best you can given the resources you've had up until now.
- You can get through this. I will help you.
- You are beautiful inside and out.
- You are perfect in this moment as you continue to move

toward wholeness and self-acceptance.

- You are in the exact right place that you need to be right now. Everything is as it should be.
- You deserve to relax.

This next part can be very challenging so please do let your support system know that you will be doing this. Call them before you do it and after to discuss.

Let your gaze fall onto your body. Notice what it looks like without judgment. No unkind words or thoughts. If judgments come in, notice them, notice how they feel. But don't dwell on them or let them take over. Be with what is real. What is real is only you. Your thoughts and judgments are subjective. For example, you might look in the mirror and notice that you have cellulite on your thighs. What is real is, "I have cellulite on my thighs." That's the only thing that's real. The thought or judgment is, "I have gross cellulite on my thighs." Inserting the word "gross" there creates a judgment. It is what it is. At this moment, try to accept what you see. It doesn't mean that you have to love it, or even like it or embrace it. But can you look at yourself without hating yourself? Can you look at yourself and accept what is there in the moment? Accepting yourself does not mean that you won't change. In fact, it's the opposite. Acceptance creates consciousness and gives you more space as well as more power to change. Some affirmations to tell yourself as you look at your body:

- My body deserves love.
- My body has gone through a lot and continues to carry me through; for that I am grateful.
- I need to treat my body with love and respect.
- My body doesn't hurt me, but I have the power to hurt my body. I am choosing not to hurt my body.
- My body is a gift and deserves to be treated with love and kindness.

- I choose to help my body stay healthy by nurturing it and nourishing it with self-love, healthy food and healthy exercise.

The point is to find self-acceptance and let go of what you believe other people think of you. Allow yourself to be accepting to yourself and others. In doing this you have so much more power. You can't control how other people are going to perceive you or react to you. It has nothing to do with you; it is in their hands. However, you can control how you perceive yourself and you can control your own reactions. In doing this, you embrace your power.

Step Thirteen – Retroflecting

Retroflection is a term borrowed from Gestalt Therapy. In nature, retroflection is the movement of an ocean current that doubles back on itself. In the human mind, retroflection is an action that was once directed towards the environment but was turned back against oneself. When you retroflect, you are hurting yourself when you really want to hurt someone else. You are angry at someone but take it out on yourself instead of dealing with this person directly.

Misty, a 32-year-old patient of mine, struggled with her weight and binge eating for most of her life. She was very close to her family, and spent many weekends and had many dinners with them. However, each time she came home from a dinner, she would go to the store and have a great binge. In fact, she almost always binged after getting off the phone with her father. She was overweight and had found that throughout several attempts of weight loss programs and weight loss camps and spas and ranches and retreats, her bingeing had sabotaged her weight loss efforts. As we worked together, Misty began to discuss her father and how obsessed with appearance he was. Her parents were society people. They were very wealthy and extremely concerned with keeping up appearances. Misty explained that every time she saw her dad, he would comment on her weight or on what she was eating. She wanted so badly to please him and to have him be proud of her. As we continued to work together she realized that she didn't want to lose weight because she was angry with her father. Because he was so obsessed with façade, and how people presented, she didn't want to give him the satisfaction of having a "thin, pretty daughter." She was also quite afraid that if she lost weight, he would love her more than he did when she was overweight. "I don't think I could handle that," she told me. As we continued to work together, Misty was able to disconnect from her father's grasp a bit. She had been so desperate for his approval that she put all of her self-worth into his ideas about her. As we worked together, she decided to put some distance between herself and her family. The more distance she had from them, the more she became able to appreciate herself for who she was without the *introjected father object* (the voice of her father inside her head that she heard as her own). As she became more confident with herself, she was able to confront her father about his comments and his desire for her to be thin. As they became more communicative, she began to notice that her father was insecure. His issues with her weight had nothing to do with her, but with her father's desire to fit in. Her father didn't feel good about himself and so he was trying to please the people around him. Misty realized that her father's issues with her weight had nothing to do with her, and everything to do with him. As she began to grasp that, and as her father began to hear her more, his comments became fewer. She realized that she had to do it for herself. She did lose some weight as she stopped bingeing, but losing weight was no longer at the forefront of her mind. She became able to talk to her father directly rather than trying to hurt him by eating. By discussing things with him, Misty also reconciled that she might not ever be able to please her father because he was just so displeased with himself. With an understanding that she was no longer working to please her dad, she was able to move on with her life and do things to please herself. In fact, she even changed careers to something that she was more interested in rather than what she had previously been doing to gain the approval of Dad.

Another patient of mine, Hanna, the mother of two young boys, found herself retroflecting when things became chaotic in her household. When her boys would run around the house out of control and her husband didn't seem to notice, care or take any time out to help, she would find herself in the kitchen bingeing.

"It drowns out the noise," she would say. "It's the only thing that calms me down when the boys are so nuts." This is another example of retroflection. Hanna was frustrated with her children and angry with her husband, but rather than engaging with the boys or talking to her husband about supporting her more, she stuffed it down with food. It drowned out the feelings, the anxiety, and the anger that she felt toward her husband.

Are you binge eating because of someone else?

Exercise One: Are You Hurting Yourself When You Feel Angry at Someone Else? – *Journal Opportunity*

Think about a time when you might have reacted to someone else by binge eating. Answer the following questions:

1. Has there ever been a time when someone did something and said something that made you feel totally helpless?
2. If so, what happened? What did this person do or say?
3. How did you react emotionally? (How did you feel?)
4. How did you react behaviorally? (What actions did you carry out in reaction to this?)
5. In thinking about this situation, was there a better way that you could have behaved?

For instance, Hanna could have walked into the living room and discussed how she felt with her husband. Or she could have left her house for a few minutes to get some air. She also could have sat down where she was and breathed. Binge eating did nothing to change the situation – it only made her feel worse.

So often people eat out of a sense of powerlessness. For countless women, because everything around them feels so out of control, they find eating serves as a wonderful way to control the way they feel about a situation. Because your eating has developed as a coping mechanism, it is the quickest and the easiest thing to do to make you feel better in the moment. Most people won't even realize that they are doing it. The baby will scream, the boss will yell, the husband will be unhelpful, the dog will get an ear infection, whatever it is, you will quickly find yourself in the kitchen. It is a conditioned response that you believe is beyond your control. The truth of the matter though is that it is not beyond your control. It feels like it is, but it's not.

As we know, there are many situations that we have absolutely no control over. My patient Kristi, a 36-year-old single mother, had recently decided to go back to school to become a teacher. She continued to work full-time while she got her master's degree in the evenings. Meanwhile, her two-year-old daughter had stopped sleeping through the night and, to top it off, she was going through a wretched divorce. She was angry with her husband, she was angry that her daughter woke up every night, she was exhausted all the time and, financially, she was not doing very well. Her situation was bad. The only thing she could do to soothe herself was to sit in the kitchen at night and eat. Eating was the only thing that calmed her anxiety and enabled her to get a bit of rest before her daughter would wake up and scream for her.

Kristi and I worked together on allowing her to let go of the situation. She knew that letting go of the situation meant letting go of control. She realized that there was so much going on for her that she had absolutely no control over. So we looked at what she could control. There were a few (albeit a very few), but there were some things that she could control. First off, Kristi had been trying to get through school as quickly as possible. She had this belief that she had to finish her master's degree in two years. This was a flawed belief. She had a sense of urgency, but she didn't know why or what purpose it served. The reality of the situation was that school would certainly be there and she could take as long as she wanted. She decided to cut her course load in half. This not only saved her money, but it helped her to feel less pressure about doing homework and being in class almost every night. Letting go of that and calming down a bit actually had a trickle down effect. As Kristi's anxiety decreased and she was home more often for her daughter, her daughter began to feel safer. This resulted in her sleeping in her bed more often at night and not waking up in the middle of the night feeling scared, unsafe and crying. As for her divorce, she began to understand that there was nothing she could do to control her husband. She began avoiding his phone calls and not engaging with him. She let her attorney field all of his issues. She figured, after all, this is what she paid her lawyer for. She completely let go of dealing with the divorce and allowed it to be in the hands of her attorney so that she could concentrate on the things that mattered to her. She realized that she couldn't control her husband's actions or reactions, so she allowed herself to let go of them. She knew that she was furious with him, but she made a pact with herself not to take out her anger on him by hurting herself with food. She put a magnet with the Serenity Prayer on her refrigerator that helped her to remember that there are many things in life that she can't control. However, she could control what she chose to put in her mouth and how she chose to cope. She began to have nightly baths with lavender oil, which helped her to relax.

The Serenity Prayer:
Please grant me the serenity
To accept the things I cannot change;
The courage to change the things that I can;
And the wisdom to know the difference.

Exercise Two: Letting Go of Control of Another Person or Situation – *Journal Opportunity*

1. Name a person or situation that is currently occurring that is causing you to feel powerless, hopeless, or out of control:

2. Is there any part of this situation that you can control? How can you do that?

3. Which part do you have no control over?

4. Admitting and understanding that you have no control over this person or situation, what can you do to soothe and take care of yourself?

5. Write a letter to this person or to the situation letting them know exactly what you're feeling. Don't hold back with this letter; let everything that you feel come out. Then, allow yourself to take the letter and burn it, or even put it in a bottle and send it out to sea.

6. If you have a spiritual or faith base, send out a message to the Universe or to your higher power or to God and ask them to hold this situation for you as it is too much for you, and that you'd like to let go of it.

Meditation Time

Imagine yourself on an island with the person or situation that you feel out of control with. See yourself saying good-bye to them or to the situation; then see yourself getting into a rowboat and rowing away. You see them and you wave good-bye as you continue to row your boat away from them. They continue to get smaller and smaller as you row further and further away. You know that the person or situation still exists, yet you are allowing yourself to detach from them.

Realize that it might be beyond your power to solve or change this situation, so make a pact that you are going to stop trying. Instead, do something for yourself that feels good – detract attention from the person or situation and put that attention on yourself.

Focus on what you do have control over and the power that you do have. Make a list of these things as well as a list of things that you are grateful for. You will never be happy if you continue to focus and obsess on the things that you cannot control. Try to refocus your energy on things that you can control. For some people that means taking up a new hobby. A patient of mine who was very sick with bulimia discovered that she had a real talent for sewing. She began making baby clothes; and in having the power to create things, she found more strength in being able to give up control of situations that she was unable to control.

Step Fourteen – Dealing with Self-Sabotage

For many women, dieting and weight loss are part of their everyday vocabulary. They spend years and even decades on diets, obsessing about them constantly. This is really a very typical binge eater, someone who diets constantly yet is always sabotaging themselves by bingeing and undoing their efforts. Let's look at this closely. Besides the typical reasons that people break their diets (hunger, boredom, hopelessness) there are several reasons why people self-sabotage and binge.

Cynthia, a 30-year-old patient of mine, had been obese since the age of 15 and had been on a diet for the past 15 years. She'd tried everything to lose the weight, including a very serious lap band surgery procedure. She'd actually managed to put on weight after getting her lap band. The more we discussed it, the more she realized that she was terrified to be thin. Cynthia was 13 years old when she began being molested by her father's work associate. He did this to her several times, yet she'd never told anyone about it, not even her parents. She was so ashamed. She thought that she had done something wrong and shameful and that her parents would be angry with her. After the first incident, she began eating for comfort and to shut out the event. Around the same time she began putting on weight, her perpetrator was arrested for molesting another child and put in jail. Even though the abuse ending had no connection to Cynthia's weight gain, she had a belief that continuing to put weight on would keep her safe. So, as an adult, trying to lose weight became impossible for her. Every time she started to lose weight, she would panic and begin to binge again. When she did the lap band surgery, there was a real chance that she'd finally lose the weight and so she did everything she possibly could to prevent weight loss. She said that she couldn't stop eating because "food is the only thing that gives me joy." She was sabotaging her own health by continuing to binge. As she began to deal with her past abuse and process through it, she started to see that food did not make her happy, but it fulfilled a great need in her. It helped distract her from the pain she was in and, on some level, she believed that it kept her safe from sexual assault. As we began addressing her trauma history, she realized that she'd been holding onto it for so long and adding self-protective layers to prevent it from happening again. She started taking a self-defense class for women. She felt so empowered and inspired by this that she went on to work toward a black belt in martial arts. Understanding that her sexual abuse didn't define her allowed her to let go of the binge eating. After admitting it to me, she joined a group for sexual abuse survivors. She finally had a voice. She was able to speak about her experiences, her anger at her assailant and, most of all, her anger at her parents for not providing a safe environment for her, not just for her to become a victim, but also one where she didn't feel safe to tell them about what happened to her. In confronting her parents, and being able to release what she'd been holding onto for so long, she no longer felt the need to binge nightly. Her weight regulated and she is actually in school now to become a psychologist to help other women deal with their sexual trauma.

Another patient of mine Lindsay, a brilliant young woman, was in the process of applying to medical school. She had several applications to fill out as well as her MCATs to study for. She had quit her job to dedicate her full attention to all of these things, but instead of sitting down and doing them each day, she stood in front of the refrigerator and ate. As we spoke, Lindsay admitted that she was so anxious about the whole process that she couldn't even look at it. She was nervous that she wouldn't do well on her MCATs, she was nervous that she would be rejected by every school that she applied for and she'd disappoint everyone around her. She was also nervous that she *would* get into medical school. Then she'd have to be in medical school for many years. After realizing that there was so much fear around both getting in and not getting in, she understood why she sabotaged herself by procrastinating with food. If she didn't even try, then she wouldn't be rejected – or accepted! Food was a very convenient way for her to avoid all the anxiety tied up in applying to medical school. Lindsay allowed herself to let go of the outcome. She decided that she'd figure out the next step as soon as she knew what the next step was. This enabled her to get serious about her studying and her applications. After addressing what it was that was really bothering her, the binge eating began to decrease. When she would go into the kitchen to eat, she'd remember, "Okay, I'm in here because I'm anxious and scared, that's okay, but I've agreed to let go of the outcome, so I'm going to close the cabinet and go back to what I'm trying to do." She wound up doing very well on her MCATs and getting into her first choice medical school. She has sent me updates telling me how tough it is but she really feels that she's in the right place.

Exercise: How are You Self-Sabotaging by Binge Eating? – *Journal Opportunity*

1. I am afraid that if I stop binge eating:
2. I am afraid that if I don't stop binge eating:
3. Some of the ways I sabotage myself with food are by:
4. Some other ways that I sabotage myself in life are by:
5. If I stopped self-sabotaging with food, what might happen?
6. If I stopped self-sabotaging in other ways, what might happen?
7. What are some ways that I can stop myself from sabotaging my good intentions?
8. Who are some people who will help support me with my goals?

Discuss with the people above what your goals are. Of course these should be safe people. Let them know what you are working on and how you've been sabotaging. Ask them if you can be accountable to them. This does not mean that they are supposed to push you or make you do the things that you want to do; it just means that they are there to listen to your goals and to listen to what happened when you self-sabotaged.

Step Fifteen – Dealing with Procrastination

Angie, a 27-year-old high achieving patient of mine, was in her second year of law school at Stanford. Since she began school, her binge eating had increased quite a bit. She claimed that she binged because she couldn't face studying, applying to internships, or working out her funding and financial aid. She had a lot to deal with and found that the only way she could was by eating. However, it never quite worked for her. She would wake up in the morning, go to class, and when she came home, she'd have several hours where she needed to be working and studying. According to Angie, the pressure at school was crushing. Each day, when she came home intending to study, she would instead spend the first several hours in front of the refrigerator snacking and scavenging for food, or out buying food, then she would eat it in front of the TV or the computer. By the time the evening rolled around, she found that she'd achieved very little and would stay up most of the night dosing herself with coffee and caffeine pills in order to get her work done. She would then spend her days feeling heavy, lethargic, depressed and anxious. Her pattern of procrastination set up a pretty bleak existence for her. She was living on junk food and caffeine, and not enjoying school or learning.

As I said in the previous chapter, procrastination is a form of self-sabotage, and food is a very easy way to procrastinate. As Angie and I worked together, she found that the proposition of being a lawyer was very scary for her. The competition at Stanford was fierce and she realized that after graduating, she would be working even harder than she had during law school. After realizing how dark her future felt, Angie decided to take a leave of absence to figure out if law school was the right step for her. She realized how unhappy she was and how procrastinating was just a way to postpone the unhappiness, and how food filled the void. On her break, she worked for an organic farm. She really enjoyed it and stopped binge eating because she was out in the world doing something she loved and looking at food in a very different way – as a precious resource. She wound up reentering school, but not law school. She decided to move up to Washington to work toward her degree in sustainable agriculture. She doesn't regret leaving law school at all, and has been free from binge eating for several years.

Exercise: Ending Procrastination and Getting Moving – *Journal Opportunity*

1. What is something that you often find yourself procrastinating on?
2. How do you feel about this particular task?
3. How do you feel while you are doing this task?
4. How do you feel while you're thinking about this task?
5. How does food help you when you are procrastinating?
6. What are your fears about doing this task?
7. What are your fears about not doing this task?

You might notice through this exercise that the task itself feels bigger than it actually is because you've created much more out of it than the simple task that it is. For many people, paying bills is a task that they put off because either they don't have the money or they are afraid to see how much they owe. Rather than figuring out a solution to this problem (like calling the creditors and making a payment plan) they will avoid it, which then results in a big drawer full of unpaid bills, stress, more eating, more avoiding, big interest rates and poor credit reports, which then leads to more procrastinating, more eating, and bigger problems that become overwhelming.

Ways to Stop Procrastinating

1. Do the thing that you don't want to do the most first. Schedule it for the morning and do it then.

2. Give yourself a non-food reward for completing your most difficult task, such as a pedicure, a bath or calling a good friend whom you haven't spoken to in a long time.

3. Break your task down into small bite-sized pieces. Rather than looking at the whole, overwhelming task, figure out the smaller steps that you need to take and do them one by one. For instance, rather than clean your whole apartment, start by choosing one room. Once you get to that room, choose one corner. Give yourself an allotted amount of time and do just that corner; tomorrow you will do one drawer, the next day, another.

4. Explore your fear of failure. Allow yourself to understand that it is okay if you fail. Try not to think of it as a failure, but as an opportunity. If you never made any mistakes, you would never learn anything.

5. Do not demand perfection from yourself. Sometimes, the overwhelming demand that the task be done perfectly can result in paralysis, rendering you completely unable to perform the task. Aim for getting it done, not getting it done perfectly. You can always fix it later.

6. Recognize that getting things done is challenging for a lot of people, so doing it perfectly doesn't matter as much as just doing it. If you can just do it, you're 75% ahead of most people.

7. Be honest with yourself about what your priorities are. Is it more important for you to spend time with your kids than to grade papers? If so, allow yourself to enjoy some guilt-free time and then get to work later.

8. Limit the amount of time you allow yourself to procrastinate. For instance, if surfing the web or playing online

games is something that you do to procrastinate, allow yourself to do it. However, set a timer for yourself and only allow yourself to do it for 20 minutes once every two hours, or whatever time constraint you set up for yourself.

9.   Make a game out of tasks. Give yourself a point or a non-food reward system for what you get done.

10.   Block out a certain amount of time to complete projects.

11.   Make your tasks small. After completing each one, take a small relaxing break before moving onto the next. This could be stretching, yoga, a shower, a bath, a walk around the neighborhood or a check-in call to a friend.

12.   Remove distractions, especially food-based distractions, from your workspace.

13.   Set a timer for 30 minutes and just do that task for 30 minutes. When you are done, you can either choose to set a timer for another 30 minutes or do something else.

Step Sixteen – Dealing with Boredom

Genette, a 29-year-old research assistant, was a patient of mine who binged specifically out of boredom. Whenever we discussed her motivations for bingeing, she insisted that she was just bored and eating gave her something to look forward to. It was something fun to do. Genette wasn't really at a loss for things to do. She had dozens of best friends, she lived in a very exciting part of San Francisco, had hundreds of cable channels as well as books and the Internet, yet she constantly felt bored. Obviously, her boredom had very little to do with a lack of options. Boredom is more about not being able to emotionally engage in an activity. Boredom also breeds an inherent internal anxiety. Rather than sitting with that anxiety, Genette had the need to fill the space with something, usually food. Boredom is rarely just that. There is always something underneath the boredom. Something such as lethargy, depression, anxiety, discontent, a feeling of being trapped, existential angst or, as it often goes, a very deep feeling of loneliness. Many people believe that boredom is a feeling, but what it actually is, is the avoidance of feelings. As we continued, Genette admitted that she felt depressed and lonely as, one-by-one, each of her friends began getting married, having kids and living lives beyond the typical partying that they had done in their 20s. Although she was beautiful, smart, funny and interesting, Genette had not really ever had a boyfriend. As we plunged deeper into her issues around loneliness and fear of being alone, she began to see that food helped her feel less lonely. It filled her up when she felt empty and gave her something to look forward to when she went home alone each night to her fabulous apartment. As she recognized that she was eating out of loneliness, she began to make peace with her boredom. She realized that when it came, it was a cue to her that she was feeling lonely. In those moments, she would allow herself to sit with the boredom as well as the ensuing anxiety that went with it. She would sit without judgment, and without trying to make it disappear with food. She would be kind to herself and give herself words of encouragement. After a few months, she decided to give it a whirl and do some Internet dating. She found that having a goal of learning how to date and possibly learn how to be in a relationship was very helpful for her in dealing with her boredom.

Exercise: Understanding Your Boredom – *Journal Opportunity*

1. Do you ever eat out of boredom?
2. When do you find that you are the most bored?
3. If you weren't bored, what would you be thinking about? (What's underneath the boredom?)
4. Do you think that you use boredom as a substitution for anything? If so, what is that?
5. How does eating help you when you're bored?
6. How does eating when you're bored hurt you?
7. Are there other ways that you can nurture yourself when you are bored? If so, what are they?
8. Are there other things that you can look forward to besides food? If so, what are they?

Step Seventeen – Sleep Issues and Night Eating

Do you find yourself up late at night grazing through cupboards, or even waking up in the middle of the night and finding that you can't go back to sleep without eating something? If so, you might be dealing with Night Eating Syndrome (NES). Night Eating Syndrome can be one gigantic binge at night or in the middle of the night, but it is usually manifested as several episodes of grazing throughout the night. NES often corresponds with anxiety and insomnia. There are theories that for people with NES, serotonin levels decrease in the evening[11] causing snacking on heavily carbohydrate-laden foods to help the body relax and get ready for bed.

Though it's challenging, there are things that you can do to defeat night eating:

First and foremost, get your sleep in order. Prioritize regular sleep habits and getting to bed at an appropriate time to allow you 7–9 hours of sleep. If you just cannot do this, consider seeing a doctor for help.

Eat breakfast! This can help to establish healthy daytime eating patterns to ensure that blood sugar and serotonin levels remain steady throughout the day.

Establish regular eating patterns throughout the day including lunch, dinner and snacks. Some people with NES are afraid to eat normally during the day since they get most of their calories at night. The irony is, however, that if you eat during the day, you might find that you need less food in the evenings.

Before you go to sleep at night, write in a journal. Write about your day, your fears, anxiety, anger, sadness, joy, excitement, whatever, just write and move your emotions through you. Meditate on a feeling before you go to sleep at night. Write about it in your journal. For instance: *Anxious – I'm feeling anxious right* *now about going to bed, I don't want to wake up in the middle of the night and eat again. It's been going on for years and I don't know how to handle it. It sucks. I'm so angry, frustrated, and mad at my eating habits. Why can't anyone help me? Why can't I stop? I'm so mad. I'm so mad...*etc. Just let your feelings move through you before you go to sleep. Keep your journal next to your bed in case you wake up in the middle of the night. If you do, write in your journal.

When you go to sleep at night:

- Turn off all the lights and television.
- Sleep with a sleeping mask and earplugs in order to ensure deep sleep.
- Put a piece of duct tape across your bedroom door so that you don't unconsciously get up and walk to the kitchen. The tape will snap you out of your trance so that you can bring some consciousness to the choice to get up and go eat.
- Put a STOP sign on or in your refrigerator so that you can remember to think about what you're doing.
- Keep a light snack like grapes or a small sandwich in the refrigerator or next to your bed that is just for you when you wake up, just a little something that will satisfy your need to eat without creating a middle of the night binge.
- If sleep meds are not an option for you, talk to your doctor or Naturopath about taking a supplement such as melatonin, tryptophan, or 5-HTP at night to increase calmness, decrease night eating behaviors and help with sleep.

Night eating is challenging because it is so unconscious, but helping your body and mind relax while increasing consciousness of the behavior can help quell it.

Shoshana, a 28-year-old client of mine, had been dealing with night eating for several years. A huge part of her pattern was coming home from work each night, turning on the television set and grazing till it was time for her to go to sleep. She would fall asleep each night with the television on. Inevitably, she would wake up in the middle of the night and bring food into bed with her. As we worked together, she noticed that her night eating was often a barometer of what was going on in her life. When work got stressful, when her relationship was feeling rocky, she would notice that she was waking up more in the middle of the night and eating.

Establishing more rituals around her evening helped her to conquer night eating. Instead of turning on the television each night, she would come home and prepare dinner for herself, and eat it in the kitchen while listening to quiet music instead of in the living room in front of the television. Sleep became an exercise in self-care. She would spend some time doing things such as washing her face and brushing and flossing her teeth before she went to bed. Once she got to bed, she would make sure that the television was off and spend 10–30 minutes writing in her journal. She wouldn't necessarily write in long cohesive sentences; she would just write whatever she was feeling, whether it made sense or not. Sometimes she would just draw a picture or free write short stories. She found that discharging the day through this kind of release helped her to sleep more soundly. Before bed she would make sure that both the television and the lights were turned off. This helped her sleep better and often get through the night without eating episodes.

Exercise One: Battling Night Eating – *Journal Opportunity*
Each night before you go to bed, sit down with a journal and begin to write. Here are some prompts to get you started:

I think:
I need:
I feel:

Today I:
I wish that:
The worst part of my day today was:
The best part of my day today was:

Of course any free writing will do. This exercise is mostly to help you move the energy of the day out of you and reduce anxiety.

Exercise Two: Establishing Self-Care Rituals

Self-care is key in healing from any kind of addiction. Where binge eating is abandoning yourself, self-care is showing up for yourself. It is the opposite of self-rejection.

Think of several self-care rituals that feel important for you to do, such as:

Flossing your teeth
Stretching
Nail care/Manicure
Pedicure
Washing your face
Bathing/Showering
Washing and drying your hair
Putting lotion on
Meditating
Dancing
Listening to music
Drawing
Praying

What other kinds of self-care rituals would you like to engage in? Continue the list. Each night, choose a couple of self-care rituals to perform. This simple act of self-love can help you to make the space for feeling better about yourself. It can also take the place of night eating and grazing.

Step Eighteen – What Do You Binge On?

Often, people use different foods to help them process different emotions. For instance, I often see people using crunchy foods such as cereal or nuts when they are angry. The crunch helps them to feel as if they are doing something active and it helps to soothe the angry feelings. Believe it or not, your jaw is the strongest muscle in your body. Because of that, it holds all sorts of tensions and anxieties and anger. So, using your jaw to crunch on things can actually release tension. Many people with anxiety will find themselves grinding their teeth at night as well. Excessive crunching can be a way to deal with frustration. Something that you can do that is a fast and easy way to release tension is to put a pillow over your mouth and scream into it. If you aren't worried about your neighbors, then don't even bother with the pillow. Something else that you can do is massage your own jaw. Simply massage little circles around your jaw muscles while breathing into your jaw. Many people find that this is instantaneously relaxing.

I've found that people who tend to binge on hearty carbohydrates like bread or pasta are looking for a way to shut off their minds. Bingeing on simple carbohydrates is a way to manage anxiety. When we digest carbohydrates, our blood sugar levels rise, and then insulin is secreted, which lowers the blood levels of most amino acids with the exception of tryptophan – a precursor to serotonin. When there is more tryptophan than other amino acids, it enters the brain at a higher rate. The brain then produces more serotonin. Drugs such as Prozac and Wellbutrin are classified as Serotonin Reuptake Inhibitors. They prevent your serotonin levels from dropping. So, in a sense, you are self-medicating when you feed yourself simple carbohydrates to help your mood. Many people equate bingeing on non-sweet carbohydrates as searching for some kind of comfort; like crawling into a soft warm bed on a cold winter night, it provides warmth, peace and comfort.

Bingeing on sweet things such as ice cream or cake serves a similar purpose; however, it also gives you very quick energy, similar to a jolt of caffeine. Many people find that they binge on sweets in the afternoon, close to the end of their workday. Often, when people could really use a little nap, they rely on some sugar as a pick me up. Other people use it at night to put them to sleep. What goes up must come down. After the initial jolt from the sugar, your blood sugar drops, sending you into a fatigued 'out of it' state of being. Many people develop Type 2 diabetes from these excessive sugar binges. Bingeing on fatty foods like cheese and heavy meats can be a need for satiety, filling a void that seems unfillable, continually open and asking for more. Because these foods are so satiating, people will often use them to try and fill emptiness inside of them.

Exercise: Considering Your Binge Foods –
Journal Opportunity

What are your binge foods? Do you have favorites? Think about what individual purpose they might be serving. What are you feeling when you're bingeing? Are you feeling frustrated? Anxious? Do you need comfort? Love? Sweetness in your life? Are you feeling empty? Bored? Think about what you eat and how it relates to why you do what you do.

Step Nineteen – How to Soothe Yourself through Uncomfortable Feelings

As we discussed in Step Eleven, human beings are blessed with millions of different feelings and emotions. Yet, for some reason, we only let ourselves feel a few of them. Happy is an acceptable emotion, but sad, defeated, angry or lonely are not acceptable, especially for women. Many women believe that they have to show up completely fine all the time. When they don't feel "fine" they become angry with themselves and judge their emotions as good or bad. There is no such thing as good or bad feelings. Feelings just are. Any feeling that you have is valid. When you push those feelings away, you might find yourself stuffing them down with food, starving them away with dieting, distracting yourself from them by obsessing on food, a diet, your body, or running away from them with compulsive exercise. When you let yourself feel them and look at them, it's easier to deal with them. As you sit with feelings, you can begin to understand the thoughts that are provoking them. By looking closely at the thoughts that are provoking your feelings, you can sometimes find more balanced thoughts that create a shift in the way that you are feeling.

There are several ways to deal with your uncomfortable feelings. One of the most effective ways is to work with the thoughts behind the feelings. This is called Cognitive Behavioral Therapy. It is very effective at changing the thoughts behind the feelings, and thus eventually changing the feelings. A part of CBT is cognitive restructuring. This is when you change your cognitive distortions. **Cognitive distortions** are usually very exaggerated or irrational thoughts that pop into your head and stay there. There's a saying in A.A. – your mind is a dangerous neighborhood. Thoughts can become beasts and torment you. Usually these thoughts turn into larger beliefs that you begin to dwell on, thoughts that you just cannot shake. They grow inside of you and perpetuate lots of internal pain. Transforming these distortions and negative thoughts can quickly and vastly improve your mood and defeat anxiety. The process of learning to refute these distortions is called cognitive restructuring. There are several books on CBT and many therapists who specialize in teaching CBT. This is an abbreviated overview with some simple exercises that can help you change the way you think.

The following are examples of common cognitive distortions as they relate to binge eating:

1. All or Nothing Thinking: Also called polarized thinking, this is when you speak in absolutes or think of everything in black and white. You expect perfection from yourself. If you are not completely perfect, you consider yourself to be a total failure.

"I ate a piece of bread with my meal. I promised myself I wouldn't eat starch anymore. I hate myself, I might as well eat this whole basket of bread."

2. Overgeneralization: You make extreme statements that refer to an individual event.

"That person gave me a weird look. She must think I look fat. Everyone here thinks I'm a fat loser. I never do well at parties. I just need to leave here and go home and eat until I pass out."

3. Mental Filter: You find something negative in every statement or incident and dwell on it so that it distorts the whole experience.

"My co-worker told me that I looked nice today. This is the first time he's ever said anything like that to me. Does that mean I usually look bad? Maybe it's because yesterday I didn't eat so I look thinner; maybe he usually thinks that I am disgusting and fat and gross. Now I can never eat again."

4. Disqualifying the Positive: When something good happens, you reject it by qualifying it with some kind of flawed reasoning.

"I got that job, but it's because I somehow tricked them into thinking I'm something that I'm not. I'm a huge fraud. Either that or they are totally desperate because they are a horrible company and no smart person would ever work there."

5. Jumping to Conclusions: You jump to a negative conclusion about something that you have no facts to support.

"I'm not going to get into that graduate program, everyone else who applies will be smarter and more qualified than I am and they will laugh at my application."

6. Mind Reading: You believe that someone is thinking negative thoughts about you and then you act on that false belief.

"That woman I work with won't talk to me because she thinks that I'm fat. She thinks that she's better than me because she's so thin. I know that she doesn't like me. I know she thinks I'm a loser. I'm so embarrassed. Forget that bitch, I don't want to talk to her."

7. Future Tripping: You look at all the negative possibilities of the way something can turn out and come to a place where you believe that this is the only way things will go.

"If I do or say one wrong thing, no one will like me at work and I'll get fired from my job. I won't be able to pay my bills, I'll have to move out of my apartment, and I'll have to move in with my parents and they will make me miserable and I'll spend all my time binge eating and I'll never find a partner and I'll be alone forever."

8. Minimizing or Magnifying: You exaggerate the meaning of something or devalue the importance of something.

"My boyfriend calls me every morning at 8am, he didn't call this morning. He must hate me. He must be having an affair. I'll bet he's going to break up with me."

"So what if I didn't binge today. That's only one day. There are still thousands more days that I did binge and thousands more to go..."

9. Emotional Reasoning: You believe that what you are feeling reflects the way things really are regardless of the evidence to the contrary and it becomes a self-fulfilling prophecy.

"I am addicted to sugar, so if I eat this one cookie, I will eat the whole box." And then you do.

10. Should Statements: You tell yourself that you "should" or "should not" constantly. When you don't live up to what you should or should not be doing, you feel guilt and shame. You also direct should statements toward others and then feel angry and resentful toward them.

"I should have self-control. I should fit into a size 4. I should be as thin as other women I see around town."

"My best friend should call me every night. She shouldn't reject me for her new boyfriend."

11. Labeling and Mislabeling: When you or someone else makes a mistake, you attach a negative label to yourself or to the other person, usually calling them or yourself a name, labeling them or yourself something other than they really are:

For instance, you drank too much last night, your reaction: "I am the biggest loser in the world."

A woman in a parking lot takes the spot you were about to

pull into. You call her a bitch, a thief, inconsiderate, self-absorbed… etc. The truth of the matter is, she just might not have seen you and had absolutely no intention of stealing your spot.

12. Personalization: You take responsibility for a negative event that you were not responsible for.
  "My boyfriend cheated on me because I am too overweight."

Katrina, a 35-year-old patient, had terrible anxiety. She would often eat to quell her anxious thoughts. If her husband caught a cold, she would go into a panic because she was sure that he was probably dying. If her boss didn't smile at her when he passed her in the hallway, she thought for sure that she had messed up in some way and that he was going to fire her, and then she wouldn't be able to get another job and she and her children would be homeless. She would often spin out into terrible anxiety that would overtake her mind. By using some simple techniques to deal with her thoughts, she was eventually able to assuage her anxiety without using food. She realized that she catastrophized with her thoughts. She set up cataclysmic situations in her head and then lived there rather than in the reality. Of course she felt anxious most of the time because she was living in a horrific alternative reality where everything was doomed.

Exercise One: Understanding Your Automatic Thoughts and How They Affect Your Feelings – *Journal Opportunity*

When you have an overwhelming feeling, follow these step-by-step directions to help you come back to yourself. Feelings can begin to overtake you and bring you into a reality that doesn't necessarily exist. Let yourself begin by following these directions.

Example:

1. What are you feeling?
   I am feeling very anxious and also depressed.
2. On a scale from 1–10, how anxious and how depressed are you feeling?
   Anxious–10, Depressed–8.
3. What are the thoughts that are triggering these feelings?
   I was at a work party last night where I drank too much. I think that I made a fool of myself when I talked to people and maybe I said or did something that I shouldn't have. Everyone thinks that I'm totally weird and screwed up. I won't have any more friends, my boss will fire me; there is no way I can show my face at work tomorrow. I am so mortified, I want to disappear.
4. For each of these statements, what is absolutely true?
   What's absolutely true is that I drank too much and that I am mortified and want to disappear.
5. How do you know that's true?
   Because I said things that I wouldn't have said if I hadn't been drinking and I woke up with a hangover.
6. Are there any thoughts here that might not be true?
   It might not be true that I made a fool out of myself. It may not be true that I did or said anything that I shouldn't have. It might not be true that everyone thinks I'm a horrible person. It may not be true that I won't have any more friends.
7. How do you know that these thoughts might not be true?
   Because I am not a mind reader and I can't know what everyone is thinking.
8. What is a more balanced truth here?
   The truth is that I'm certainly not the first person to get drunk at an office party. In fact, I was only one of several people there who were enjoying alcoholic beverages. Very few people probably noticed whatever I said or did. In fact, I know that people are usually so anxious about what other people are

thinking of them at these functions that I imagine very few people are wasting their time obsessing over what I did or did not say. Besides, if I lose friends for one night of being a little outlandish, I will know that these weren't real friends anyway.

9. What kind of cognitive distortion was this?

    Magnification: *I blew something out of proportion. It probably wasn't as bad as I thought.*

    Should Statements: *I should never look silly or out of control.*

    Jumping to Conclusions: *No one will talk to me.*

10. How are you feeling now?

    Still anxious, yet a bit calmer. I can get up and walk away from this for now. I don't have to eat something to stuff it down and feel better.

11. On a scale from 1–10, how anxious and depressed are you feeling?

    Anxious–7, Depressed–5

Some of the worst things in my life never even happened
– Mark Twain

Many people get very carried away in their thoughts. This is one of the great causes of anxiety. They tend to ruminate on something that did or did not happen and get very carried away by thoughts that are absolutely untrue. They believe that they know what other people are thinking and have stories in their head like, "Everyone thinks I'm… a bad person… stupid… fat… ugly… a bad mother… a bad wife… needy… annoying…" etcetera. When we acknowledge our thoughts without fearfully pushing them away, we can also challenge them and find an answer that might be better.

The truth is, you can never know what another person is thinking. You also can't control what other people are thinking. Many people with eating issues try to control other people's thoughts and perceptions through controlling their own food intake. This is because when someone notices you or sees you, you absolutely lose all control. You can't control what they are seeing or perceiving or how they are going to react to it. Everyone sees through their own filters. This is what makes body image so complex. We want people to see what we want them to see or not to see. And we can't control how they interpret what they see.

Use your journal and try the exercise on your own now. You can also find the automatic thought log in Appendix F.

Think about a time when you were feeling very upset about something.

1. What are you feeling?
2. On a scale from 1–10, how strong are these feelings?
3. What are the thoughts that are triggering these feelings?
4. For each of these statements, what is absolutely true?
5. How do you know that's true?
6. Are there any thoughts here that might not be true?
7. How do you know that these thoughts might not be true?
8. What is a more balanced truth here?
9. What kind of cognitive distortion is this?
10. How are you feeling now?
11. On a scale from 1–10, how strong are these feelings now?

You can use the automatic thought log any time you are feeling caught up in your head and unable to escape from your thoughts, or any time you are just feeling distressed and needing some help out of that dangerous neighborhood.

Exercise Two: Stop Sign

When your thoughts are just out of control, try to imagine a big stop sign in your brain. You can even say it out loud: "Stop. I refuse to engage with you." You are reminding yourself here that your thoughts are invasive and probably unproductive. You are refusing to give them airtime as these intrusive thoughts have no benefit and do nothing other than hurt you.

Despite all this, there are times when you might just feel badly and no amount of looking at your thought patterns will change this. It is crucial at these times to give yourself permission to be in your feelings without shame and without judgment. The judgment creates worse feelings than you are already having. You feel badly, then you make yourself feel worse for being angry at yourself for the way you feel. This is unfair. When you are with your pain, maybe even at peace with it, the hurt and the anger and the fear and the sadness will feel less scary and you will not need to avoid it with food. It's a gift to learn to feel safe with your feelings. Talking to a good friend or a safe person can help you to sort out your feelings and not feel so alone with them.

Step Twenty – Healing Shame

Shame and eating disorders almost always go together. Shame fuels eating disorder behavior by making people believe that they are bad, worthless, defective or unlovable. Chronic shame is the constant belief that there is something intrinsically wrong with you. You aren't born feeling shame. You feel shame when the outside world treats you in a way that causes you to believe that you are unworthy.

Sidney, a 37-year-old woman with extreme binge eating behavior, grew up in a military family that valued physical fitness above all other attributes. Sidney, however, was unathletic and bookish. Instead of playing sports with the other kids at lunch, she would sit by herself and read. Unlike the other kids, she wasn't bony – she was built a little differently, more robust. She was incredibly bright and revered by all of her teachers, but her father was disappointed by her lack of athleticism. He and her mother put her on a very strict weight loss diet and mandated that she did sports after school. She was not allowed to eat the same meals as everyone else in her family. Her brother could have cookies, cake, ice cream, steak, mashed potatoes, bacon cheeseburgers, whatever he wanted! Sidney was stuck at dinner with broiled chicken and cooked spinach. There was very little variation. And although her brother didn't do half as well in school as she did, because he was slim and trim and did well at sports, their parents gave him more praise and admiration, while Sidney just got punished with a diet. So unfair! It led Sidney to feel extremely ashamed of herself. She hated herself because she couldn't excel in sports and she hated herself for the kind of body she had. Since her parents only let her eat broiled chicken and cooked spinach, she began to steal food and eat in private, which then intensified her shame. She started eating out of the garbage can at school – all the leftover Twinkies and Ho Hos she could ever want! Unfortunately, when she was caught she was sent to the principal's office and suspended. Sidney needed help, she was suffering immensely; but instead of finding her help, she was punished by her parents. This just perpetuated her feeling of being bad. She believed that she was a bad person both for who she was, and for who she wasn't. She was bad because she had a bit more padding than other kids her age and she was bad because she wasn't a sports fanatic. These values weren't placed upon Sidney by herself; they were imposed upon her by her family. She was perfectly content with her body and loved to read. But she was taught that neither were okay. She believed that she was fat, ugly and disgusting. But she wasn't. She recently brought pictures into our session from when she was a little girl. She wasn't fat at all. In fact, she looked like a normal little kid. However, at that age, she believed that she was obese. As she got older, her sneak eating increased. Eventually she became a full on binge eater – dieting by day, and bingeing alone at night. By the age of 37, her weight had become a problem for her. Not only that, but she was still eating out of the garbage both at home and at work. She was jeopardizing her job and her marriage wasn't being tended to because she was so obsessed with food and with dieting. She had a great deal of shame about her size, her shape and the fact that she didn't play tennis or go running with the other mothers in the area. All of her old shame still sat with her. She really believed that just because she was a woman of size that there was something wrong with her. She believed that people didn't like her, and that she had to go above and beyond for each person because she felt so inherently unlovable.

As we worked together, Sidney realized that these beliefs did not belong to her. These came from growing up in a military family who valued physical fitness above academic endeavors. As she began to understand that she was just different from them, and that her values were just as important, she became okay with who she was and her life began to improve. Rather than trying to keep up with the sporty moms, she found a group of women who did a biweekly book club. She joined a writers' group and started spending time with people whose values more closely resembled hers. After she stopped comparing herself to people who had completely different philosophies on life, she stopped feeling so ashamed for who she was not and was able to more easily embrace who she was. As she liked herself more and grew close to friends who liked her for who she was rather than how she presented, she stopped obsessing on dieting, calories and exercise. As the obsessions began to fall off, the bingeing minimized and she finally began to accept that her body was more solid and larger than the pixies that she'd been aspiring to look like for all those years. She found that she could embrace who she inherently was rather than be ashamed.

The antidote to shame is acceptance. Shame comes from outside of us. It is triggered by people, institutions, society, or ideas that teach us or treat us in such a way that we come to believe that we are not worthwhile or loveable as we are. Looking at the people around you and noticing whom you are choosing to surround yourself with is a great first step. Are the people around you loving and accepting or are they shaming and punishing? Do they accept you for who you are or do they want you to be someone else? Part of recovering from shame is surrounding yourself with people who are supportive, safe and consistent. This doesn't mean that you need to surround yourself with people who are constantly flattering and complimenting you. That's not safe or honest either. However, it is important to find folks who reflect back to you the essence of who you are and see you for all your positive attributes, and love and accept those. When you surround yourself with those who are consistently criticizing you or somehow leading you to feel inferior, you will notice that it is difficult for you to feel good about yourself. You will constantly feel "not good enough, not smart enough, not pretty enough..."

and on and on. Some people believe that it's important to surround themselves with people like that in order to really know 'the truth' about themselves and where they have to improve. This is a myth. The truth is subjective. Why is it that someone who looks down on you is any more right or intelligent than someone who sees your positive traits and likes you for those?

Exercise One: Breaking Away from Shaming Friends or Acquaintances – *Journal Opportunity*

1. Make a list of people whom you feel either inferior to or badly about yourself when you are around them.
2. Who are some people that you like yourself when you're around?
3. What reasons do you have for spending time with the first list of people?
4. What are some ways that you can create limits with the first group of people and increase your time with the second group?

Spend time around people that you like, but spend more time with people who you like yourself the most around. When you spend time with people who bring out your best traits, you will find that you like yourself better more of the time. This is most important when it comes to your partner or spouse.

Exercise Two: Understanding Your Family Patterns of Shame – *Journal Opportunity*

Growing up with shaming parents, it is easy to fall into the trap of spending time with shaming friends. However, you have that choice now. You are not beholden to them.

Parents, however, no matter whether or not they are estranged or passed on, stay with you forever. Ponder the following questions in your journal.

1. Did you or do you feel badly about yourself around your parents?

2. What things did your parents say or do to cause you to feel badly about yourself?

3. How are these things still with you?

4. Your parents probably held these beliefs and acted this way because:

5. Just because these messages came from your parents, does that necessarily mean that they are true? Why or why not?

6. Is it okay for you to make the choice not to accept this shaming message?

7. What are some new, non-shaming messages that you can integrate into your psyche?

8. What are some ways that you can allow yourself to feel these new messages?

Those are ways to begin to understand how external messages can contribute to internal feelings of shame. In order to challenge your internal manifestations of shame you must identify the underlying beliefs that cause you to feel that shame.

Exercise Three: Challenging Omniscient Internal Shame – *Journal Opportunity*

Below are some common self-limiting thoughts that perpetuate shame. Check those that apply to you and explore where this belief came from. Then, in your journal write your own challenge statement. There is an example after each one. You can use that one, or you can write one that is more pertinent to your situation.

1. Self-Limiting Thought: I must always be doing something, I am nothing if I am not constantly productive
This belief states that you are valuable for what you do, not for who you are. You believe that your job performance, your

grades, the amount of money that you make is what gives you value. It is not okay for you to be a human being, you must always be a human "doing."

Do you have this belief? If so, what do you think led you to believe this?

When do you first remember feeling this way?

Shameful Belief: Being productive is what gives me value.

Challenge Statement: The person I am is already valuable.

- What are some other positive beliefs you might have?
- How can you practice and integrate the positive beliefs?

2. Self-Limiting Thought: I must always be perfect

Perfectionists believe that if they are anything less than perfect, that they are not okay. One of the challenging things about being a perfectionist is that it makes it very difficult to learn and enjoy new things. Many perfectionists won't even try to do something new if they don't think that they're going to be good at it the first time – and let's face it, no one is good at anything the first time. So, many perfectionists miss out on trying new games or sports, or dating, or learning to dance, or learning a new musical instrument, or learning to knit or to sew and on and on. The truth is, even the master yogis and yoginis had their very first day of yoga class. Like anyone on their first day, they walked into that yoga studio scared and alone amongst people who were way ahead of them in practice. Even the most talented pianists had to sit down and learn to play do-re-mi. You are not born with an innate knowledge of how to do everything; you have to be willing to try and to learn. No one is ever perfect when they first try something, but that is okay. Taking risks enriches your world.

Do you have this belief? If so, what do you think led you to believe this?

When do you first remember feeling this way?

How have your food issues and body image issues played in to this belief?

Shameful Belief: I always have to be perfect no matter what.

Challenge Statement: I am a human being, with perfectly human flaws. I make mistakes sometimes and that is okay.

- What are some other positive beliefs you might have?
- How can you practice and integrate the positive beliefs?

3. Self-Limiting Thought: I never do anything right

Many people who had parents who told them such things as "you'll never go far in life," or "you're nothing but a screw-up and that's all you're ever going to be" or "you always mess up, can you never do the right thing" grow up into adults who believe that they are worthless. These kinds of statements are not only painful and damaging to a child, but they are also very untrue. When someone says "you always..." or "you never..." it comes from a very young, immature place. Intact adults know that superlatives are rarely founded. A parent who has said these things to you is most likely repeating something that he or she heard in their youth. It's untrue that things "never" work out for you. It's untrue that you "always" mess up. This is the cognitive distortion polarized thinking, which is very self-limiting and even more so when it comes to food. The thoughts, "I'll never stop bingeing, I'll never eat like a normal person, I'll never like my body, I will always be fat..." are deep-seated beliefs that come from years of frustration and the shame of not believing that you can achieve what you want to achieve. This is about not believing that you have what you need inside of you to be who you want to be. This is just untrue. Few things in human nature are absolutes. You have everything you need inside of you to live the kind of life that you want to live. You have to realize though that these old beliefs are nothing but flawed beliefs.

Do you have this belief? If so, what do you think led you to believe this?

When do you first remember feeling this way?

How have your food issues and body image issues played in to this belief?

Shameful Belief: I can only fantasize about what I want; in real life though, things don't ever go my way.

Challenge Statement: I create my own destiny and I have the power to do what I want to do; the only person who has the power to stop me is me. I am choosing to go forward, not stop myself.

- What are some other positive beliefs you might have?
- How can you practice and integrate the positive beliefs?
- When you think about your eating issues, what defeating thoughts do you have?
- What are some ways to challenge these defeating thoughts?

4. Self-Limiting Thought: I have to be smaller, stronger, faster and smarter than everyone. Nothing less is acceptable.

This is super common among people with eating issues. The belief is that you always have to be better and do better than everyone else and you always have to beat out everyone around you to be okay. You are also constantly competing with yourself and others and trying to be better and better and better. This belief just tends to perpetuate itself. "I can't like myself until I reach this goal… okay, I've reached this goal. Can I like myself now? No, you have to do this now…" This comes from the belief that you are not enough and that you constantly have to be more. There is nothing wrong with setting and achieving goals; however, if you don't love and accept yourself until these goals are completed, will you ever be allowed to like yourself? Wouldn't it be nice to like yourself and achieve goals simultaneously?

Do you have this belief? If so, what do you think led you to believe this?

When do you first remember feeling this way?

How are your overachieving beliefs tied in with food and your body?

Shameful Belief: I am not doing enough, I have to do more, do better and be the best.

Challenge Statement: I am doing what I can and allowing myself to enjoy myself and my life while I am doing it.

- What are some other positive beliefs you might have? How can you practice and integrate the positive beliefs?
- What are some ways that you can balance liking and nurturing yourself while still being goal-oriented?

5. Self-Limiting Thought: I am a worthless human being

This is the belief that you are totally worthless. You are not good enough, you are not smart enough, you are not pretty enough, you are not thin enough, you don't have enough money... You believe that your feelings don't count, you believe that your needs don't matter, that other people's needs should always come before yours, that you should always sacrifice yourself for the sake of others. You believe that what you say is trivial or insignificant, that your input is not valuable or intelligent, that you can't contribute to a conversation. You believe that what you do in the world isn't enough or isn't valuable. This comes from a lack of love, validation and affirmation. Many people who feel unworthy put all their self-worth into caring for others. They believe that if they don't, they are unacceptable. They get their self-worth from making sure that other people are okay while avoiding themselves and not tending to their own needs.

Do you have this belief? If so, what do you think led you to believe this?

When do you first remember feeling this way?

How have your food issues and body image issues played in to this belief?

Shameful Belief: Who I am is not very important. In order for me to be valid, I have to make sure that I am doing things for other people constantly. If not, I'm worthless.

Challenge Statement: I am a worthwhile person just because of who I am. I don't have to give all of myself to people in order to be valid in the world.

• What are some other positive beliefs you might have?

• How can you practice and integrate the positive beliefs?

• There are some great things that I do appreciate most about myself. Like:

6. Self-Limiting Thought: I am responsible for everything and everyone around me

This is the person who makes sure that everyone at a party is having a good time. You believe that if things go wrong it is your job to take care of everyone and everything. If someone is having trouble, it's your responsibility to fix it for them. For many people, this comes from being a part of a family where parents were constantly blaming while choosing not to take any responsibility for their own actions. For instance, a parent who has lost their temper and then abused their child either physically or emotionally then blames the child for provoking them to lose their temper. This child grows up feeling responsible for the reactions of everyone around them. They are hypervigilant, always making sure that they are completely aware of the dynamics of every situation that they are in and the subtle nuances of people's mood changes. If they are with a person who becomes moody, upset or angry, they personalize it, believing that they are the cause of it and that they must ameliorate it.

Do you have this belief? If so, what do you think led you

to believe this?

When do you first remember feeling this way?

Shameful Belief: I always have to be in control of the situation and make sure that I am taking care of everyone and everything.

Challenge Statement: I am not responsible for anyone's actions or reactions except for my own. I only have to deal with my own emotions and allow space for each person to take care of themselves.

• What are some other positive beliefs you might have?

• How can you practice and integrate the positive beliefs?

• These are the people and situations that I am always trying to control:

• I understand that these things are beyond my control and I am willing to let go of them by doing the following:

7. Self-Limiting Thought: It's not okay for me to set boundaries

This is the person who cannot say "no" to anyone. She feels that she has no right to personal space. She owes people things, such as sex, help, money, or explanations and justifications for her behaviors, thoughts or feelings. When you don't know how to set boundaries, you often feel guilty for saying no to people. The problem is you often feel resentful of those people whom you should have said no to. Saying "no" doesn't make you a bad person. It is okay to be a self-advocate. In fact, it's crucial that you look out for yourself first. If you spend all your time taking care of others, where are you? You've left yourself to be there for others, but you need to be there for yourself. Part of that is learning to say "no" to people.

Do you have this belief? If so, what do you think led you to believe this?

When do you first remember feeling this way?

How have your food issues and body image issues played

in to this belief?

Shameful Belief: I have no choice than to do whatever you want or need me to do.

Challenge Statement: My life is my own. It is my responsibility and my right to say "no" and to do whatever feels safe for me, no matter what it is.

• What are some other positive beliefs you might have?
• How can you practice and integrate the positive beliefs?
• Who are some of the people and/or situations in your life that you need to say "no" to or set boundaries with?

The next time someone asks you to do something, ask yourself the following question: "If I don't do this will I feel guilty? If I do this will I feel resentful?" If the answer is yes, this is probably a good opportunity for you to try to set boundaries and say "no" or come up with a mutually beneficial compromise. There are of course times when you will say yes and want to do what the other person asks you for. There will also be times when you don't want to say yes but, for certain circumstances, you have obligations that you must follow through on. For instance, you have obligations to your children, or sick family members or friends or for someone who has also been generous with her time and energy. It's important to understand the law of reciprocity here. Allow yourself to give, but also to receive. If you are the only one giving, there is no balance.

• Are there places in your life where the balance should be restored? Where?
• How can you make that change?
• How have food and your body been unbalanced? How can you change that?

8. Self-Limiting Thought: I am a slacker

This is the belief that your life is out of your control and you have no ability to make it better. You feel that everything is a certain way and there's nothing you can do to change it. You are stuck in your circumstances. This is a result of dwelling on your failures in life and not celebrating or recognizing your successes. This often comes from parents who punish their children for doing something wrong, but never reward them for doing something right. There is no positive reinforcement. Thus, the failures are louder and more prominent in your mind, so much so that you don't remember or believe that there was a time that you ever did succeed. It is okay to fail. As I've stated before, if you never made any mistakes, you would never learn anything; but you have to persevere in order to move forward in your life. This goes especially for binge eating. It's easy to backslide and have a binge, but what can you learn from the slipup?

Do you have this belief? If so, what do you think led you to believe this?

How does this belief about yourself relate to food and your body image?

When do you first remember feeling this way?

Shameful Belief: I have no ability to improve my life.

Challenge Statement: I have the power to create the life that I want for myself. I am not powerless. I am capable and strong.

- What are some other positive beliefs you might have?
- How can you practice and integrate the positive beliefs?
- What are some of the failures that you've had?
- How can you apply this to food and your body?
- What are some accomplishments that you've had?
- What are some things in your life that you've always wanted to do that you've always been too afraid of?

9. Self-Limiting Thought: Everyone should like me

People-pleasing behavior comes from the belief that all others must like and approve of you and that you are only acceptable if everyone likes you. This comes from receiving love or support that was conditional, for example, "I love you when you get good grades" or "I love you when you are thin." It also comes from being neglected and only receiving praise when what you do benefits someone else. For instance, your parents ignore you until you begin to do things around the house like cleaning and doing laundry; then they give you praise. It makes you believe that you are only valid when you have the approval of people outside of yourself. There is an inability to find validation within.

Do you have this belief? If so, what do you think led you to believe this?

When do you first remember feeling this way?

How does this relate to food and your body image?

Shameful Belief: I need to do whatever I can to please people around me.

Challenge Statement: I am fine just the way I am even if some people don't like or approve of me. Liking myself is what matters the most. I don't need other people to tell me whether or not it's okay to do that.

What are some other positive beliefs you might have?

How can you practice and integrate the positive beliefs?

For each person who loves and adores the President, or a popular musician, or a famous actor, there is a person out there who despises that person. The disapproval of the public doesn't make these people any better or worse at what they do or who they are. If we all worried so much about what other people thought of us, we'd all be paralyzed because we just cannot please everyone, we just cannot make everyone like us. It's a daunting task because it's impossible. You can't control other people's thoughts and actions, just your own. Love yourself first. You are the only one who can know for sure how you feel about yourself.

Something that I like about myself or want to do more of, that other people might not like or approve of, is:

- What might happen if I did these things that certain people in my life did not approve of?
- What are some ways that I can get support and deal with that?

10. Self-Limiting Thought: I am terrified that people will leave me or reject me

This fear of abandonment comes from the belief that people will leave you because you are not worthy of love. This is a result of receiving love inconsistently. Being neglected, rejected, abandoned or just not being seen or heard by the people closest to you can make you wonder whether or not you are actually valued and cared about. This can make you question whether or not you will be abandoned again. This can also be the result of a situation, such as a parent dying when you are young, or a parent abandoning you either intentionally or unintentionally, or a single parent being stressed out with trying to make ends meet and unable to give you the attention that you need. As an adult, this can lead to you carrying out unconscious acts in such a way to test people to see if they are paying attention to you or noticing you. It also might be a way for you to figure out whether or not they will leave you.

Do you have this belief? If so, what do you think led you to believe this?

When do you first remember feeling this way?

Shameful Belief: People will inevitably abandon me and I will always be alone.

Challenge Statement: I am perfect, whole and complete exactly as I am. People want to be around me and won't abandon me.

- What are some other positive beliefs you might have?
- How can you practice and integrate the positive beliefs?
- Are there people in your life who are rejecting and

abandoning? Who are they?

- Is it necessary for you to keep working to ensure that these people will stay with you?
- Why or why not?
- Are there some people in your life who you feel safe and secure with?
- How do you know that they won't abandon you?
- What are some ways that they have led you to believe that they are not planning on abandoning you?

11. Self-Limiting Thought: Conflict is not okay and I must avoid it at all costs

You believe that it's not okay for you to ever speak up for yourself or disagree no matter what you think about the situation. Conflict avoidance comes from being in a family where feelings or situations were ignored or glossed over. Everything was always fine, even if it wasn't. This leads to insecurity because you believe that it's not okay for you to express your feelings open and honestly. It leads to binge eating when you stuff down feelings rather than talk about them.

Do you have this belief? If so, what do you think led you to believe this?

When do you first remember feeling this way?

Shameful Belief: I should keep my mouth shut no matter how I'm feeling about a situation.

Challenge Statement: My thoughts and feelings are valid and important, and it's okay for me to talk about things that bother me open and honestly.

- What are some other positive beliefs you might have?
- How can you practice and integrate the positive beliefs?
- What are some conflicts that you try to avoid?
- Do you ever use food to push down your feelings when you avoid conflict? If so, how?
- What might happen if you didn't avoid these conflicts?

12. Self-Limiting Thought: People can't know who I really am or the things I really think about or do

This is the belief that if people really knew who you were, they would reject you. This is also the fear that your coping mechanisms (i.e. binge eating) will be discovered and your cover blown. The belief is that you have to hide your authentic self and project a false self, that you should be ashamed of who you really are and must act fake in order to be okay in the world. This is a cover-up. Usually people who project a false image have grown up in a family where there were secrets. Things such as sexual or physical abuse, alcoholism, suicide, eating disorders, or mental illness weren't spoken about. Issues were ignored or avoided. This causes a false projected self and a false sense of self. So not only are you projecting a fake you out onto the world, but you are also rejecting your own feelings and believing that there are certain things that it's not okay for you to feel.

Do you have this belief? If so, what do you think led you to believe this?

When do you first remember feeling this way?

Shameful Belief: It's not okay for me to be having these feelings. My feelings are wrong. People can't think that I have feelings such as sadness, anger or loneliness. People can't know the shameful things I do to cope with these feelings.

Challenge Statement: It's normal and human for me to have varying ranges of emotions, thoughts, habits and coping mechanisms. Everyone does and it is okay for people to see the real me. I don't have to use unhealthy coping mechanisms or be alone with this; I can get support and help from others out there dealing with similar issues.

What are some other positive beliefs you might have?

How can you practice and integrate the positive beliefs?

Doing these sorts of behaviors leads to a complete rejection of self. There is so much fear that people will reject you for who you really are that you head them off at the pass by rejecting yourself first. This way, presenting a false image becomes self-protective. "If people reject me, they're not really rejecting me, because I wasn't real." It is a way to keep you from being vulnerable. However, it also keeps you from being in real authentic relationships. When you are presenting a false self, you are in a false relationship with someone. As you begin to allow yourself to know the real you and you allow people to get to know the real you, you will find that your relationships are deeper, stronger and more fulfilling.

- What are some ways that you reject your true self?
- How can you practice accepting your true self?
- What would it be like to start showing people who you really are?
- Is there anything that scares you about doing that? If so, what is it?
- What would be the possible negative consequences of showing people your true authentic self?
- What would be the possible positive consequences of showing people your true authentic self?

13. Self-Limiting Thought: I don't have any needs

This is the belief that it's not okay for you to have needs or to let other people know that you have needs. You never believe that it's okay for you to come first. You might completely ignore your own needs in order to tend to the needs of others. This might come from watching a mother who rejected her own needs for the sake of the family and shamed you for having needs. You might have been told that it's not okay to whine, to be sick, to be needy.

Do you have this belief? If so, what do you think led you to believe this?

When do you first remember feeling this way?

Shameful Belief: It is never okay for me to have any needs, if I do I am needy. I have to be completely fine all the time.

Challenge Statement: Human beings are interdependent. We all have needs and it's okay for me to express those needs and trust that there are certain people who will meet them.

- What are some other positive beliefs you might have?
- How can you practice and integrate the positive beliefs?
- What kinds of needs do you have that you feel unsafe expressing?
- Do you ever suppress your need for food in order to feel better or more virtuous?
- What unmet needs have you been suppressing?
- Who do you feel safe expressing your needs to?
- How can you start to do this?

14. Self-Limiting Thought: I am a total loser

This is the self-critical/self-hating belief that you are no good. This can be a result of physical, emotional, mental or sexual abuse. It can also come from the inability to manage or control your life successfully. People who feel this way have a tape in their head that is continually telling them that there is something wrong with them.

Do you have this belief? If so, what do you think led you to believe this?

When do you first remember feeling this way?

Shameful Belief: It's not okay for me to be me. I have to change in order to be okay.

Challenge Statement: I am fine the way I am. I'm just fine. As long as I am a kind human being and hold myself with integrity, I know that I'll be okay. I don't have to be anything other than the great person that I am.

- What are some other positive beliefs you might have?
- How can you practice and integrate the positive beliefs?
- What are some things that you like about yourself?

- What makes you valuable as a human being?
- Who believes in you and cherishes you?
- How can you start to internalize their voice of love for yourself?

Step Twenty-One – Dealing with Your Inner Critic and Gaining Self-Esteem

Earlier, we discussed the voice of the inner critic. The mean voice inside your head that says things like, "Don't say the wrong thing, everyone will think that you're stupid," or "You look really fat in those jeans", "Those people are laughing at you", "That girl thinks you look fat", "Your skin is a mess", "You can't go out looking like that", that's your critic. That is the *driving voice* of your eating disorder.

Laney, a 37-year-old patient of mine, had been struggling with binge eating since she was just eight years old. She remembers coming home after school and eating bowl after bowl of Honey Nut Cheerios. Laney was the only child of a single struggling schoolteacher mom. Her mother worked hard for them to live in an upscale neighborhood. After her day of work, she waited tables at a nearby restaurant and Laney stayed home alone. Because they didn't have the same kind of money that the other families in their neighborhood had, Laney often came to school in hand-me-downs, and without the latest fashion trends. Her mother worked hard to pay the rent so that she could put Laney in a good school in a good district. However, she was frequently ostracized in school and made fun of because she looked different. Each afternoon, tired, lonely and depressed, Laney would put cartoons on and eat cereal alone until her mother came home. After a full day of work, plus an evening of work, her mom often came home angry, stressed out and tired. She would scream at Laney for lying on the floor, being lazy and not doing her homework. She would tell Laney that she sacrificed and slaved away every day so that Laney could have a good education and there she was, ungrateful, just sitting around being lazy, watching TV and not doing her homework. Her mom said that she needed to work hard, that she had to compete with all the other kids in her school and do better than them because without being the best, she was nothing, just an ordinary person who wouldn't go anywhere in life. As you can imagine, this was probably not the best way to get Laney motivated. As she grew up, Laney kept the belief that she was a loser, a nothing unless she achieved greatness. Every single day, from the moment she woke up, she vowed to be perfect in every way. She tried to have a perfect body, she tried to be perfect at work, she tried to be a perfect friend. But no matter what she did, she felt as though it wasn't enough. She had gone to a good college, and gotten a great job. She worked in a high-level sales position and brought in millions of dollars in revenue for her company each quarter. Although her days were spent with a fake smile plastered on her face, when she came home from work, she succumbed to her secret shame. She would make two to three boxes of pasta and wash them down with a bottle of wine while completely zoning out in front of the television. No one would ever expect this from such a well-groomed, high functioning woman. Laney was the President of the Perfect People's Club. But inside, she felt so much anxiety and pressure to always be perfect that she needed a way to blow off some steam and stop the internal voices from criticizing her. They always told her that she had to be better, that she wasn't good enough, that everyone had to like her, that everyone had to think that she looked great, that she was easygoing, that she was smart, that she was never in a bad mood. She had to be super human! And she worked really hard to keep this appearance up. The problem was, she was never ever happy. No matter what she achieved, how she looked, how many promotions she got, how much money she made, she still couldn't find peace. She was so keyed up all the time, that she was never able to stop and enjoy her achievements.

Inside of Laney lived a very loud critic. This critic was constantly telling her to lose weight, to work out harder, to stay at work later, to do more for everyone.

When we began working together, Laney couldn't conceptualize the critical voice as an entity that she could separate from herself. She believed that it was just a part of her, and if she let it go she would have no motivation to do anything. She'd become a "fat blob on the couch with no job and no money." She really believed that without this 'motivation' from the harsh stories that she told herself she would collapse. She felt that talking to herself in harsh tones was the only way that she got things done.

Many people have come into my office asking me to help them attain self-esteem. Self-esteem isn't some kind of magical force whereupon you suddenly have it and you're a completely different person who loves themselves completely, stands tall and glows. No, you don't achieve self-esteem. It is more subtle than that. Healing isn't about actively changing who you are to make yourself acceptable; it's about accepting who you *already* are. When you love and accept who you are, change happens naturally. Self-esteem is not about what you gain, it is what you lose. Letting go of the negative and punishing thoughts that you have about yourself is the first step in feeling self-worth. Self-esteem is subtle. It's about being okay with who you are and loving yourself enough to recognize your faults and flaws and be able to accept them so that you can lovingly change them. Laney believed that if she accepted herself, flaws and all, she would never change. Acceptance doesn't mean being resigned to being a certain way; it means recognizing and acknowledging what is real. When you accept it without putting a judgment on it, you then have the power to change it. For example, each week, Laney came in crying and so ashamed and angry at herself about her evening pasta parties. She kept saying over and over again, "I'm so disgusting, this is so bad, why can't I stop!? I'm so gross..." and more things like that. We worked on not putting a label on her bingeing, not good, not bad, it just is. Eventually she was able to come in and say, "I binged again last night. I accept that I have a problem with binge eating. It's so difficult and I'm struggling. I don't like doing it because I feel uncomfortable and sick afterwards. I'm so tired of waking up at 5am each morning to go to the gym and work off my binges from the night before. Bingeing is really negatively impacting my life." This is a very different statement than, "I am disgusting and I hate myself and why can't I stop doing this?" When she was able to accept what she was doing without putting a judgment on it, she gained the power and the strength to change it. Acceptance is empowering. When you accept what is real without judgment, you have the strength to get out from under it. Self-flagellation turns you into both the victim and the perpetrator. You are victimizing yourself when you call yourself cruel names and berate yourself for doing things that you don't want to. This puts you in a very difficult position and weakens you. You then become trapped as both the person who is being abused (the victim), as well as being the abuser (the perpetrator). As you continue to victimize yourself, you fall prey to continuing your behaviors because you are too weak to get from under them.

Imagine your critic as an evil dictator riding on your back and holding a whip to beat you with as you move through life. Now imagine that you are in a race up the side of a mountain with someone who lacks an inner critic. You begin racing up that mountain side-by-side. Your critic is weighing upon you, whipping you and demanding that you go faster and faster. The guy next to you, with no critic sitting on his back, is just kind of walking along, stopping, smelling flowers, enjoying his stroll up the mountain. Who gets to the top of the mountain first? We don't know. But what we do know is that by the time you get to the top, you're too tired and beaten down to enjoy the view.

Laney's evening binges were a refuge from her loud, overbearing critic. After a full day of submitting to its oppressive, overwhelming commands and demands, she needed to numb out and relax. Wine and pasta helped her to completely escape not just from her stressful day, but also from herself.

As she began to fight against her critic and become strong enough to stand up to it, she realized that this was an old survival mechanism. Her mother had told her that unless she was better than everyone else, she was nothing. She wanted her mother's approval and worked hard to get it. She also felt that she was completely irrelevant without the approval from those around her. She worked her ass off to constantly have the approval from her peers to the detriment of herself. When she finally began to give herself approval, she found that she needed it less from those around her. She was able to relax more and enjoy the view rather than fighting so hard.

Exercise One: Meeting the Inner Critic – *Journal Opportunity*

At the beginning of healing your critic, you might find it too challenging to confront your critic or to challenge it. That's okay. Start off slowly just by acknowledging it and separating it. For a couple of days, each time your critic says something to you, write it down.

Example:

Date & Time: *2/14 8:30am*
Event or Trigger (what happened): *I was trying to get dressed in the morning and couldn't find anything to wear.*
What My Critic Said: *You look fat and ugly in all your clothes, everyone is going to feel sorry for you because you're single on Valentine's Day. Everything you put on makes you look like a pink pig. You might as well stay home and eat chocolate all day long.*
How that Made Me Feel: *I felt miserable and powerless and anxious because I had to get to work but I was paralyzed. I couldn't do anything.*
How I Reacted or Behaved in Reaction to This: *I lay on the floor and cried and wound up getting into work 20 minutes late.*

It's in these times that acknowledging your critic and realizing that this is the voice of your eating disorder can be liberating. Just because that voice is there doesn't mean you have to follow it. It's the same as eating a whole box of Girl Scout Cookies. Just because you have the overwhelming urge to eat the whole thing doesn't mean you have to follow it. Recovery isn't necessarily about getting rid of these urges or these voices, but about acknowledging them and not giving them too much power. Name the voice of your critic. I had a patient who called her critic "Mrs. Dartmouth". When she heard Mrs. Dartmouth criticizing her, she became able to say, "There goes Mrs. Dartmouth with her crazy yelling again." Eventually the voice began to lose its power because she was no longer engaging with it in the way she once had. You can hear the voice, but you don't have to listen to it. Acknowledging it is not about listening to it; it's actually about separating it from yourself. For instance, when you hear sirens outside your window, you are not listening to them; you are hearing them, but not actively engaging. When you hear the critical voice, you can hear it like background noise and not actively engage. Once you are able to externalize it, it can then be something separate from you, background noise. You can then choose not to let it have control over you. You can imagine these voices like dandelion seeds dancing through your mind. They're just words, thoughts, feelings, old beliefs that you can watch fly by; but you don't have to allow them to take root and grow. You don't have to water them and let them grow and flourish.

Try to spend a few days separating yourself from the critic. Use the following prompts to begin to understand more about how your critic comes to you and tries to hurt you. The worksheet is also available in Appendix F or online.

Date & Time:
Event or Trigger (what happened):

What My Critic Said:

How that Made Me Feel:

How I Reacted or Behaved in Reaction to This:

Exercise Two: Getting to Know Your Critic –
Journal Opportunity

Now that you've met your inner critic, let's get to know who this is. Begin by taking some space in your journal to draw a picture of your Inner Critic; you can also color, sculpt, sketch or paint your critic. Then, give your critic a name. Next, explore the following prompts in your journal:

I find (name of inner critic) _____ helpful because:

I am afraid of letting go of _____ because:

A positive result of letting go of _____ might be:

This is how I imagine I might feel if I let go of _____ :

Something that _____ often tells me is:

The first time I heard this criticism was from **this person** _____ during **this situation** _____ :

My mother often criticized me: True or False

If so, how?

My father often criticized me: True or False

If so, how?

My mother often criticized herself or others: True or False

If so, how?

My father often criticized himself or others: True or False

If so, how?

My mother often criticized my father: True or False

If so, how?

My father often criticized my mother: True or False

If so, how?

One very critical person I remember being around was:

They often did or said this:

Those critical voices who are not yours, that stay with you and become your own voice, are called your critical introjects. You have taken on someone else's critical voice and allowed it to become your own voice. Now, it's time to separate that voice out. No child is born hating him or herself; this is something they are taught to do, whether intentionally or unintentionally.

Take one day and notice every time your critic says something negative to you. Write down the time of day and what the critic has told you. Some people are surprised and find that their critic is with them more often than they thought. The point of this exercise is not to dwell on the things that your critic says to you, but to see the critic clearly so that when you hear these voices you can begin to distinguish that you don't have to own the voice.

Example:

7:20am: *Your pores are disgusting today. You can't go out looking like that.*

7:22am: *You ate too much last night, you are bloated and disgusting today.*

7:40am: *Why did you order that Danish? You don't need all that sugar and fat.*

8:15am: *The way you said good morning to your boss sounded weird and fake, he probably noticed.*

Notice how often your critic shows up. You need to create something in there to fight for you. That's when your nurturer and your cheerleader show up. By giving them voices, you have ammunition against your critic, and are able to stop your critical voice from taking over your mind. Because the inner critic is so pervasive, sometimes it feels impossible not to buckle under its crushing weight. When you create your own inner nurturer, you will have someone who will fight with your critic and care for you when your critic is beating you up. Your critic might begin to see that she needs to be nurtured too. As you and your critic allow nurturing to come, you might find a softening that you didn't know existed within you. You also need an inner cheerleader, someone who encourages you, energizes you and cheers you on, someone who motivates you positively rather than by berating you.

Exercise Three: Learning to Talk to Your Inner Critic – *Journal Opportunity*

First, assemble your army by taking some space in your journal to draw a picture of your Inner Nurturer; you can also color, sculpt, sketch or paint your nurturer. Then, give your nurturer a name. Next, explore the following in your journal:

What does your inner nurturer mean to you? How can he/she help you?

Next, draw, color, sculpt, sketch or paint your Inner Cheerleader:

What does your inner cheerleader mean to you? How can he/she help you?

Now that you know who lives inside of you, all the many faces of your critic, nurturer and cheerleader, you can begin to fight your critic.

Answer the following prompts in your journal.

If I overeat, my critic says to me:
If I had one, my inner nurturer would then respond:
If I had one, my inner cheerleader would encourage me by
 saying:
If I think that I've said something stupid, my critic tells me:
If I had one, my inner nurturer would then respond:
If I had one, my inner cheerleader would encourage me by
 saying:
If I have hurt someone's feelings, my critic tells me:
If I had one, my inner nurturer would then respond:
If I had one, my inner cheerleader would encourage me by

saying:

If I make a mistake at work or in school, my critic says to me:

If I had one, my inner nurturer would then respond:

If I had one, my inner cheerleader would encourage me by saying:

If I notice that I have put on some weight, my critic says to me:

If I had one, my inner nurturer would then respond:

If I had one, my inner cheerleader would encourage me by saying:

If I accidentally overdraw my bank account, my critic says to me:

If I had one, my inner nurturer would then respond:

If I had one, my inner cheerleader would encourage me by saying:

Once you are able to separate your critical voice from yourself and externalize it, by making it an entity separate from yourself, you can begin to talk back to it. Talking back to your critic is empowering. It gives you the ability to not get so engulfed by the negative thoughts in your head, and enables you to bring yourself back.

Example:

Critic: You are walking down the street and you hear a group of men or women laughing. Your first thought is that they are laughing at you. This is not real; this is your critic making up stories. How do you respond to your critic?

Your Response: I'm not so self-centered as to imagine that everyone walking down the street is paying attention to me. Of course they aren't laughing at me. They probably didn't even notice me walk by. And if for some reason they did and they are laughing at me, there surely must be something wrong with them, not with me because what kind of a person laughs at someone when they are walking down the street? Not a very nice one.

Critic: You look fat and ugly today. You shouldn't leave the house. Stay in bed all day today and do nothing. No one should be forced to look at you.

Your Response: You can't talk to me that way. I don't look very different than the way I did yesterday. I am fine. I might be unhappy about something totally different and I am taking it out on the way I look. I might have binged last night, but I am still me. Rather than making myself feel worse by berating myself, I'm going to take extra special care of myself today.

Now, in your journal, create some responses for other things that your critic might say to you.

Critic: Don't talk; if you do, surely you will say the wrong thing and everyone will think that you are stupid.

Your Response:

Critic: You fat pig, you better not eat anything today.

Your Response:

Critic: No one will ever want to date you until you lose the weight.

Your Response:

Critic: You have one month until that wedding, you need to lose 20 pounds in that time. What crash diet can you go on?

Your Response:

Critic: You are not smart or good-looking enough to spend time with those people.

Your Response:

What other kinds of things does your critic tell you? How can you then respond? In your journal, begin to keep track of the kinds of things that your critic says and how you would like to respond to it.

As much as your critic torments you, you might also be projecting your inner critic onto other people. Do you find yourself judging other people's choices or actions? Do you often think things like, "I can't believe she did that, I would never do that!" Many times, when people have a harsh inner critic, they tend to compare themselves to others in order to judge how they're doing in the world. For example, "Am I prettier than her? Am I smarter than her? Am I thinner than her?" Some people need to feel superior to others in order to feel good about themselves. However, putting people down in order to elevate yourself gives you a fake sense of grandiosity. You're not actually elevating yourself; you're just looking down on people so you feel elevated. What you might practice is sending positive thoughts toward those around you. It just feels different in your body to let go of the negativity. When you do, you are naturally elevated. Letting go of your critic allows you to feel better about both yourself and others.

Your critic might seem like a large overpowering judge. But it is really a child. A weak, scared, sad child – who is afraid of being hurt, who is afraid of being abandoned, who is afraid of being criticized, who just wants to protect him or herself, so it tries to act big and scary. It becomes a monster. But when you remove its scary monster uniform, you will discover that it's just a frightened little girl or boy.

Step Twenty-Two – Being Kind to Yourself

When recovering from an eating disorder or any kind of addiction, learning to take incredibly good care of yourself is paramount. Up until this point, you've taken care of yourself with food, or believed that you weren't good enough or deserving of being taken care of – everyone else was more important, others' well-being came before your own. Now it's your turn. Taking care of yourself comes first. Of course that can be so hard for someone who doesn't feel self-love. It becomes a vicious cycle.

"I binged/drank/used drugs/acted out sexually and I hate myself, I must punish myself, I don't deserve anything good. I have to hide..." It's a good idea to start by just doing the things that you need to do for basic self-care; for instance, go to the dentist, get your annual physical exam, take your vitamins, floss your teeth, shower daily, get your hair cut... things that you need to maintain and care for your body. After those basic things, you might want to think about more self-loving things, such as getting a massage or a facial or going on a retreat.

Sometimes the idea of doing self-loving behaviors feels not just overwhelming but unauthentic and fake. One way to deal with that is to begin to consistently check in with self-inquiry, "If I loved myself, what choice would I make?"

Sometimes you will be confronted with a giant box of cookies. Part of you might say to eat the whole box, another part of you might say to not let yourself have any, another part of you might say just have one or two, while another part of you tells you that if you have one or two, you won't be able to stop. Ask yourself, "If I loved myself, what choice would I make?" And begin to meditate on that. Perhaps the part of you that loves yourself realizes that it's not the right time for you to have any cookies as they might trigger a binge, or it might tell you to go ahead and take two and put the rest in the freezer for later or to give them away. This is about using mindfulness and self-love to change your behaviors. Although you might not inherently feel self-love, there is a part of you that loves you unconditionally. There is a part of you that doesn't care if you binge or if you purge, if you're fat or if you're thin. This part of you doesn't care if you say something stupid or if you stumble or if you embarrass yourself. This part of you loves you and wants you to thrive and to be happy. Although that part might be so quiet that you can barely hear her, she is there. You might have to find her though. When you ask the question, "What would I do if I loved myself?" you give that part of you a voice. Eventually she gets louder and takes over your critic.

Exercise: Positive Affirmations

Positive affirmations are declarations or positive statements that are made to practice the art of positive thinking. Affirmations have gotten a lot of flack as being new agey or silly. They conjure up images of Al Franken's character Stuart Smalley on *Saturday Night Live* repeating his affirmation, "I'm Good Enough, I'm Smart Enough, and Doggone It, People Like Me!"

For many people, affirmations feel very forced and untrue and saying them does very little. For affirmations to work, you have to believe them somewhat.

Jana, a 28-year-old nurse, was told by her 12-step sponsor to stand in front of the mirror naked every day and look at herself, and say over and over again, "You are beautiful and perfect just the way you are." Jana didn't believe it and the affirmations themselves wound up doing more harm than good. Although she was saying this wonderful affirmation to herself every day, she felt disgusting inside and did not believe what she was telling herself. This set up an internal conflict because although she was telling herself out loud that she was perfect and beautiful, inside she was telling herself: "Bullshit, you are disgusting and fat and ugly." Each day she left for work in a terrible mood. As we began to work on her daily affirmations, we decided a few things. First off, she didn't have to be naked in front of the mirror; it was too triggering and shaming for her. She also didn't have to say anything that she didn't mean. Instead of saying things that she didn't believe, she created some affirmations that she did believe. She began to look at herself in the mirror in the morning and say, "Your body deserves to be loved and taken care of, no matter what it looks like," and she believed it. She wrote down several affirmations on index cards and pulled them out when she needed them, or looked at them in the morning as she brushed her teeth. As she continued to believe that her body did deserve love, she eventually began to see herself as beautiful. Only then did she begin to believe her original affirmation.

Think about things that you might not believe but would like to believe about yourself. Create affirmations that would help you achieve these feelings. Write these affirmations on index cards and carry them around with you in your purse each day to look at them when you are feeling down on yourself or when your critic is loud. Place them on your bathroom mirror, or on your work computer.

Affirmations should make movement. They should not cause you to stop and have an internal conflict with yourself. Using affirmations should help you to get to your eventual goal. But you need to make sure that you actually believe the affirmations that you are making. For example:

The Goal You Want to Accomplish	The Affirmation to Help You Get There	The Eventual Affirmation
I don't want to hate my body any more.	My body deserves love.	I love my body unconditionally, just the way it is.

I want to stop binge eating.	Each day I am working on reducing my binge eating. Sometimes I slip up, but that's okay, it's a normal part of the recovery process.	I am completely at peace with food.
I want to be perfect.	It's okay for me to allow myself to be human. Part of being perfectly human is being imperfect and I can accept that.	I am perfect, whole and complete just the way I am.
I want everyone to like me.	Some people will like me and some people won't. That's okay, I know that I am a good person and that's what counts.	I love myself completely.
I want to lose weight.	I am working toward having a healthier body. As I continue to make healthy choices, my body will settle into its natural weight.	Food nurtures me and keeps my body healthy and beautiful.

In Appendix F or online, find your own sheet for creating your affirmations.

Step Twenty-Three – Letting Go of Polarized Thinking

In Step Nineteen, we learned about cognitive distortions. Polarized thinking, which is also known as all or nothing thinking or black and white thinking, is a cognitive distortion that is very common for binge eaters.

Polarized thinking is an extreme sort of thinking, when you have rigid beliefs about certain things where there is no room for compromise. This is the belief that something is all good or all bad. This rigidity can be around people or objects or situations; but often, when the polarized thinking is about food, it leads to extreme behaviors around food and body image and it also leads to binge episodes.

Latisha, a 32-year-old woman, had the rule for herself that she should run on the treadmill for one hour daily and eat no more than 1200 calories each day. If for some reason she couldn't get her run in, she would spend the whole day bingeing or conversely, if she went above her calorie count at all, even by 20 or 30 calories, she would skip the gym and go home to binge for the rest of the night. Because her rules were so rigid, there was absolutely no room for any flexibility in the day or week. If she was unable to abide by these rules, she felt that the day was ruined and she'd just begin again tomorrow. This is an extreme example of all or nothing thinking. In her quest to gain complete control and domination of her behavior, Latisha actually had no control at all.

When you see yourself in this way, there is very little peace within. You are either forcing yourself to fit into a very tight mold or berating yourself for not being able to maintain that behavior. All or nothing thinkers are either on a diet or off a diet. There is no room for healthy eating with occasional treats. You are either good or you are bad. If you are not perfect, you are a total failure.

There is no middle ground. Latisha and I first worked on helping her to allow herself to lighten up a bit on her exercise routine. Rather than running on the treadmill each day for an hour, she would hit the gym 2–3 times a week for vigorous exercise for 30–45 minutes; and the rest of the week, she would exercise more gently. For example she would do yoga, or take a stroll or a light hike with her iPod, or even go out dancing. At first it was very challenging for her. A walk or a yoga class barely seemed like exercise to her. As she began to allow herself to enjoy her strolls and her yoga classes, she began to integrate the peacefulness within that she had been looking for with her severe food and exercise patterns. She had believed that the sense of control helped her feel at peace; when in fact, it actually caused more inner turmoil. The next goal was for her not to binge on the days that she didn't run. Because she wasn't running, she believed the day was a wash, so she might as well binge. She began to understand how distorted that thinking was. Just because she didn't run it meant she had to binge? Absolutely not! That wasn't helpful. As she let herself stop bingeing on the weekdays, she began to also allow some more calories into her day. At first it was impossible for her not to count calories. She agreed to up her calories slowly. Week by week we would increase her calories by 100. She eventually got up to 1800 calories per day and at that point noticed that her urges to binge were lessened. She eventually even allowed herself to eat more on the days she was exercising vigorously. Ironically enough, despite everything she believed about dieting and exercise, she began to steadily lose weight. She came to her natural weight after a few months without bingeing and compulsive exercising. She finally understood what I meant by "trust your body to tell you what it needs." Eventually, as she gained body trust, she was able to stop counting calories, and with that, her binge eating decreased dramatically. She has maintained a stable weight for several years and has gained a sense of peace that comes from feeling safe around food.

Although she was petrified, Latisha faced her fears about integrating flexibility into her rules. She tentatively trusted me and then allowed herself to surrender to body trust.

Trying to be so 'good' all the time is a desperate attempt to avoid being 'bad'. However, good and bad are subjective. Eating a cinnamon roll doesn't make you bad any more than eating a salad makes you good. As you know, restricting food eventually causes a binge, and excessive exercise leads to pain, burnout, injury and a distaste with exercise that causes one to avoid exercise altogether.

When you first decide to let go of your binge eating, all or nothing thinking can often interfere. This is because this sort of thinking doesn't hold the reality that progress is not linear. It wants to be perfect in recovery as well. However, recovery is not perfect; it is a learning process that takes time, and often includes relapses that enable us to learn from them. If we binge, even a mini-binge, or even if we are able to stop ourselves from continuing a binge that we have already started, the all or nothing thinking won't allow us to congratulate ourselves on the progress. It will tell you that you are a failure and that you'll never get over this. As you begin to integrate flexibility, you will see each small step as great progress and be able to accept that you are not perfect; you are a wonderful work in progress and hopefully you will be for the rest of your life.

Notice your language. Do you say things like, "I *always* fail" or "He *never* puts away the dishes" or "You're *always* late"? When you speak or think about yourself or others in absolutes, you're coming from a very young, self-protected space. Adults know that life and people are not all or nothing. However, children don't understand that, and believe that events or people are completely one way or the other in order to stay safe. This helps them discern where to go, where not to go, what to say, what not to say, and generally helps them understand the rules of life. This way of seeing the world is a psychological defense called splitting. It is useful and important when you are young, but as you get older and have the ability to look at events and situations from different vantage points, and see the pros and cons and sort through all the different possibilities of a situation, you realize that splitting doesn't always serve you. Notice when you begin to go into these forms of thinking. You might be going into a regressive state where you are scared and trying to keep yourself safe.

Just like anything new, Flexible Thinking (instead of all or nothing thinking) may be uncomfortable at first. However, after spending some time in the middle of the road getting used to being perfectly imperfect, the journey becomes much easier and more enjoyable.

Letting go of all or nothing thinking and integrating flexibility can be scary and challenging.

Exercise One: Integrating Flexible Thinking – *Journal Opportunity*

Try to imagine some flexible thinking options for each scenario:

1. You are at a restaurant with a friend and you vow not to eat any bread. However, the dinner rolls come out and, despite your best efforts to restrain yourself, you wind up eating one.
   What is the all or nothing thinking?
   What are some flexible thinking options?
2. You are planning on wearing a particular pair of pants to a party. However, on the night of the party, you realize that the pants feel a bit too tight.
   What is the all or nothing thinking?
   What are some flexible thinking options?
3. You go to a party and decide not to drink any alcohol that night. However, you give in eventually and have a glass of wine.

What is the all or nothing thinking?

What are some flexible thinking options?

4. Your friend is late for your dinner date and you are sitting alone in a restaurant.

   What is the all or nothing thinking?

   What are some flexible thinking options?

5. You have gone to the store and charged a sweater on your credit card after vowing that you wouldn't rack up any more credit card debt.

   What is the all or nothing thinking?

   What are some flexible thinking options?

6. You have vowed not to eat any sweets for one month. After a few days in, you find yourself eating some cake at a birthday party.

   What is the all or nothing thinking?

   What are some flexible thinking options?

7. You decide to go to the gym every single day. One day, you wake up late and don't make it.

   What is the all or nothing thinking?

   What are some flexible thinking options?

8. You have decided that you can only eat 1500 calories a day. At the end of the day, you add up your calories on the Internet and find that you've eaten closer to 2000 calories.

   What is the all or nothing thinking?

   What are some flexible thinking options?

9. You get into a very big fight with your partner or spouse or a close friend. You are incredibly angry with this person.

   What is the all or nothing thinking?

   What are some flexible thinking options?

10. You have made a decision to make wholesome healthy choices and to practice good nutrition. You are at a restaurant and you order what looks like the healthiest

option on the menu, fish tacos. However, when you receive your meal, you find that the fish is completely breaded and fried.

What is the all or nothing thinking?

What are some flexible thinking options?

It is always good to remember that you have options. Everything isn't so black and white. There are always grey areas. You might think that there are only two choices. However, it's important to notice when you might not be giving yourself all the available options. When confronted with a situation that seems hopeless, as if there is only one option, take time to stop, breathe, think about your options or create new options that will be stronger than simply settling for whatever is in front of you or your default choice. It is always within your power to create new options for yourself.

Exercise Two: One Daily Intention

When your thinking is so black and white, you might wake up every morning vowing to be perfect. By 10am, that vow might already be broken thus creating the compulsion to act out considerably since your eating disorder is telling you that *it's the very last time…*

Rather than being perfect, just make one daily intention when you wake up in the morning. These intentions can be pretty simple, for instance:

I will meditate once *just for* today

I will choose to withhold judgment from myself and others *just for* today

I will eat mindfully *just for* today

I will drink eight glasses of water *just for* today

I will walk on my lunch break *just for* today

I will choose to exercise responsibly *just for* today

I will smile at five new people *just for* today
I will go to a yoga class *just for* today
I will eat vegetables with two meals *just for* today
I will not overeat *just for* today
I will be extra kind to my partner *just for* today
I will not eat in my car *just for* today
I will not use laxatives or purge *just for* today
I will take my dog on an extra long walk *just for* today
I will make my bed this morning *just for* today
I will choose not to engage with my inner critic *just for* today

What other kinds of daily intentions can you make? Make just one, and write it down in the morning. Keep it in your pocket or in your purse or wallet and look at it every so often. One thing per day can help to raise your self-esteem significantly. As you continue this exercise you might find that you are able to do two or more things each day. You might even find that you are able to keep these intentions for multiple days as you eventually begin to mold new behaviors for yourself.

Step Twenty-Four – Releasing Your Fear of the Binge Food

This step is done specifically to teach you how to let go of the belief that you cannot stop once you start. Doing this exercise several times will actually change your brain.

Diane, a 34-year-old woman, believed that once she started eating chocolate, she would not be able to stop until whatever she was eating was gone. Unfortunately, she had the problem of consistently bingeing on chocolate. During a session that we had during the spring, I asked her to bring in one of her binge foods. What she brought was a bag of Cadbury Mini Eggs.

"These do it to me every time!" she told me. "Someone keeps them in the office and I can't have just one or two; I have to eat until the bowl is gone. It's so embarrassing. I always have to run out to Walgreens to refill the office bowl."

She brought them in a small plastic bag. There were about a cup of them in the bag.

"How many do you think is an appropriate serving for you?" I asked her.

"Maybe about five," she said.

"Okay, take five out of the bag and put them in your hand." She looked at me suspiciously. This was not an easy exercise. Diane was letting me in on a very intimate moment; she was with her binge food, her lover, the thing that gave her comfort and safety and I was intruding in their space. She took five mini eggs out of the bag and put them in her hand.

"Now," I said, "take one and smell it." She held it up to her nose.

"What are you feeling?" I asked her

"Angry at you. You're staring at me and judging me and you're invading my private space. I want to eat this right now. But I feel like you're not letting me."

Anger is not an uncommon sensation when someone begins

226

engaging in mindful eating. Depression is said to be anger turned inward. Many of us believe that it's not okay to be angry. We push anger down with food and turn it in on ourselves. It becomes depression, inner turmoil, pain, and self-loathing. When we stop eating mindlessly and using food to push the anger down, it begins to surface and that is very uncomfortable.

"It's okay for you to be angry, Diane. Do you know what you're angry about?"

"I'm angry that you aren't letting me eat this."

"Anything else?"

"I had a crappy day at work today."

"What happened?"

"My boss yelled at me for something I didn't do, and I just sat there and took it, accepted her rage because there is no use in defending myself. I'll just come off looking bad."

"So now you want to crunch down on these chocolate candies and let all the rage melt away."

"I guess," she told me.

"Okay, Diane, go ahead and close your eyes. I will close my eyes too so you don't feel that I am watching you eat, and just take one bite of the egg."

We both closed our eyes as I heard her crunch down.

"Now as you chew," I told her, "chew slowly. Notice the feeling of the candy in your mouth. Notice the tastes on your tongue. Notice the thoughts and emotions that come up for you. Let me know after you swallow, but don't take another bite."

"Okay, I swallowed," she told me.

"What did you notice?" I asked her.

"Well," she said, "it was funny. Even though I was eating and tasting my food, I just wanted to hurry up and swallow so I could take another bite and keep eating. I was barely able to enjoy what I was eating because I just wanted to chase the taste. I just wanted more."

"What do you think about that?" I asked her.

"It's definitely interesting," she said.

"Okay, go ahead and close your eyes, and finish the candy."

We both closed our eyes and she put the rest of the candy in her mouth. She chewed slowly and swallowed.

"What came up for you?" I asked her.

"Well," she said, "I started thinking about my Aunt Meryl. Every Easter she would have an Easter Egg hunt for us kids. Me and all my cousins would spend the day outside playing and running around and looking for eggs. The days had just started getting longer and I knew that summer was around the corner. We would play until dusk then sit around and have a gigantic Easter feast. Of course then, it took my father forever to get me into the house to eat. Back then I loved to play... now, it's all about the food... now I'd be waiting impatiently for the food to be served. Anyway, back then I just loved being away from my dad and my stepmother's house. My aunt was so warm and loving. I loved to play with my cousins. Then she'd send me home with a giant Easter basket, back to the lonely dysfunction of my dad's house. I'd sit alone in my room sad that the day was over. The candy in my basket gave me comfort."

Diane realized at that moment how much her food and her eating were connected to her feelings. I asked her to take another egg, close her eyes, and put it in her mouth. As she did, I reminded her to really taste it in her mouth, feel the texture on her tongue, the flavors on her taste buds and the sensations of chewing on her jaw and in her teeth. After she swallowed, she opened her eyes and said, "It didn't taste that great."

"What do you mean?" I asked her.

"Well, it wasn't really anything. I feel like I'd go ahead and keep eating to try and recreate the first bite, but when I really pay attention, I didn't really need any more than the initial bite to receive the pleasure. Anything after that, I was just chasing the flavor."

I asked her if she wanted any more. "No," she said, "I'm good for now."

"Okay," I told her, "why don't you take the remaining three candies and bring them home with you for dessert this evening. Remember to eat them slow and notice what happens while you eat."

We then made a plan for what she would do for the rest of the night to avoid a binge. She planned to go home, make herself a healthy dinner, eat the remaining candies slowly for dessert, and then take a bath before bed. She left the big baggie full of candies in my office and took home just the remaining three.

One of the primary thoughts that go through a binge eater's mind when they come in contact with their trigger food is, "Once I start, I can't stop." Which is another reason why trigger foods activate a binge. Many binge eaters will be able to eat something normally and in moderate amounts in front of people, but will then go home and binge on it in private. Elena, a 28-year-old mother of five-year-old twins, was often complemented on her figure. She worked hard to keep herself looking svelte. She exercised daily and stayed far away from sweets. She believed that if she started on the sweets, she wouldn't be able to stop. When she brought her kids to birthday parties, she would always say, "Just a small slice," and that is all she would eat at the birthday party. However, on her way home, she would stop off at the market and buy a whole birthday cake and eat it alone in the kitchen where her husband and kids couldn't see her. That's not unusual behavior for someone with binge eating issues. Many patients describe going out and having a lovely meal with friends where they split a decadent dessert. Even though they've only shared half of the dessert in front of someone, they will still go home and binge. They believe they cannot stop, so they don't. The most common behavior is someone buying a box of cookies and although they've promised themselves that they'd only eat 2 or 3, they won't stop eating until the cookies are completely gone.

The truth is, you probably can stop. That's why this exercise is important. It will prove to you that you can actually stop a binge before it starts. Eating a few cookies is not a binge. Eating 30 cookies is. With this exercise, you will change your brain. You brain currently thinks that you can't stop. Unless someone is force-feeding you your binge food, you can stop. The belief that you cannot stop is just that, a belief.

Exercise: Eating Trigger Foods without Bingeing

Because this exercise is so intense, please wait to do it until you feel ready, when you are feeling courageous in your recovery. This might be after a month; it might be after a year.

Make sure to do this exercise with either a supportive friend or a therapist.

1. Before you get your trigger food, make a plan as to what you are going to do after the exercise is over to avoid bingeing.

    If you have your support person with you, make plans to spend the rest of the day or evening doing something with them such as watching a movie, going for a walk or a hike, or doing something else that does not revolve around food. If you choose to do this with your therapist, make a safety plan with him or her as to how you are going to take care of yourself after the session. If you do it alone, think about taking a walk, a bath or a shower, watching a movie, calling a friend, writing in your journal, going to a yoga class, meditating, or doing things that are soothing to you.

2. Think of a food that historically you've believed that you've not been able to stop eating or one that has triggered a binge.

3. Go out and buy a package of that food. Try to buy a one serving size portion of the food. If that is not possible and

if you are planning on doing this alone, while you are in the store take a portion (whatever you believe a portion size to be; if you don't know, look on the label) and put it in a bag. Give the rest of the food to either the person who rings you up, or someone who might be looking for food. If you are unable to do this, throw the rest out. Though it is not ideal to waste food, there is no difference if it was wasted by disposing of it or by bingeing on it.

4. Bring the food home or to your therapist's office. If you are not alone, ask your therapist or friend to close their eyes with you. If you are with someone, have them lead you through the following directions. Otherwise, answer the following questions in your journal.

    1) Take one item of food from its packaging and smell it. What feelings does the smell evoke?

    2) Close your eyes and take one bite. Chew the food very slowly. Notice the way the food tastes on your taste buds, notice how it feels in your mouth, notice what your jaw feels like as it crunches down, notice the texture of the food and how your teeth feel chewing it.

    • As you concentrate on the sensation of eating, what emotions do you notice you are feeling?
    • What thoughts or memories are coming up for you?
    • What physical sensations are being triggered?
    • What emotions are you feeling?

    3) Take another bite of the food. Chew it slowly and feel it in your mouth. Really taste it. Sense it. Tune in to your feelings. Notice what is going on in your body, your somatic response. Does your body feel excited? Tingly? Overstimulated? Shut down? Think about what your reaction to the food is. Are you triggered to eat more? Do you like the taste of it? What does it remind you of? What does this food mean to you?

4) Think about how much more you would like to eat, but make sure that you don't finish it all; even if there is one bite left over, let yourself leave some. Allow yourself to continue eating slowly, very slowly and mindfully with your eyes closed, really focusing on the tastes and the feelings evoked.

When you are ready to stop eating, leave the remainder of the food with your therapist or give it to your friend to leave with. Do not be left alone with the binge food no matter what. Make a plan with your therapist or friend as to what you are going to do for the rest of the day to avoid bingeing. Just because you've eaten the binge food does not mean that you have to binge. You are not unsafe in your body. You are strong and you have free will. This food is not stronger than you are; the need to binge is not stronger than you are. Each time you are able to eat a trigger food and not binge on it, you decrease your risk of binge eating, you reduce the charge of the food and the hold that it has over you and you assert your personal power over bingeing. It becomes easier as time goes on and you eventually find that you can learn how to eat certain foods in moderation. Repeat this exercise several times until the 'charge' of the food decreases. Discuss with your friend, therapist or write in your journal about what you notice your relationship to this binge food is.

Step Twenty-Five – Learning to Love Your Body

One of the most pervasive symptoms that accompany Binge Eating Disorder is hatred of one's body. In fact, this body hatred can often precede the eating disorder.

Hatred of your body is learned but it's not your fault. Unfortunately, we are taught in this society to worship a skinny body. A skinny body represents not just what it is, skinny; it is thought to represent self-control, self-esteem, virtue, intelligence, wealth, being healthy, being calm and cool, having it all together and being desirable. It also represents youth, naïveté, innocent sexuality, vulnerability, and sexual power – the ability to say no. The media and popular culture has a bad habit of portraying people of size to be emotionally unstable, poverty stricken, lacking self-control, having poor self-esteem, being loud, being undesirable, being jealous, greedy, needy, wanting more, being too much, being unhealthy, being unworthy and being sexually available.

These assumptions are of course not consistent or thought by everyone; however, they are perpetuated in the media and in society with fat jokes, comedy at the expense of someone's size, and insults. It's disgusting and it's wrong, but it exists. And because it exists, it is challenging for many women who exist in a body that is larger than the societal ideal. It is also challenging for women who have bodies that meet the ideal. It is a feminist issue and it's a societal issue. Female bodies are exploited. They're exploited for lust, for sex, for advertising, for humor and for the sake of exploitation. Michelle Obama is a brilliant attorney yet she is famous for being the First Lady with the best biceps. Janet Reno, the former Attorney General, was constantly berated for her less than trendy style. During the 2008 Presidential Election, Sarah Palin, the Vice Presidential

Candidate, was referred to as a VPILF and had photoshopped bikini pictures of herself all over the Internet. So, yes, it is hard to be a woman. As women, we are constantly being told that our worth is tied up in the way we look, in how tight our thighs are and how large our breasts are. And so then, we spend years, lifetimes even, eating, dieting, dieting, bingeing, dieting, purging, exercising, dieting, bingeing, crying, starving, running, lifting, taking potions and pills, smoking, snorting, drinking, stuffing, restricting... it's exhausting, and it's not even our problem. Yes, that's right, your weight is not your problem; it's a problem of society. We, unfortunately, live in a time where women are judged by the size of their waists rather than by the size of their hearts and their brains. We can't change the times that we live in. However, we can refuse to participate. We can only waste so much time, so much of ourselves trying to fit into a mold that someone else wants to stuff us into. We will never fit into that mold. We can, however, be who we want to be. We can learn to enjoy ourselves in the body we have. We can participate in sports or outdoor activities, we can play music, we can write books and stories, we can cook, we can love, we can travel. We can do anything. But we can't wait until we are the right size. You are right, right now. If you wait, you might have to wait forever.

My own mother at 5'2" weighed 112 pounds. She was terribly unhappy with that weight. More than anything, she wanted to weigh 108 pounds. From the time that I was cognizant of my mother, I remember her war with those four pounds. Each morning, she would step on the scale and curse at it. She tried and tried and tried to lose those four pounds. Over the years I remember several different kinds of exercise equipment in and out of our apartment. She ordered things off the television almost every month that would guarantee that she could lose the extra pounds. Our apartment was littered with As Seen on TV equipment. We had abdominimizers, thighmasters, cellutrimmers; we had every videotape and weight loss plan that Richard

Simmons ever touted. We had diet books and plans all over the bookshelves. We were vegan, we were macrobiotic, we did the lemon, cayenne, maple syrup fast back in the mid-90s. But no matter what she did, she couldn't lose those four pounds. It was an obsession that she died with. At fifty-four years old, my mother died of an autoimmune disease that ravaged her whole body. She died at 80 pounds. All those years had been spent trying to reach a number. When she eventually did, it was because she was sick and dying. I miss her terribly.

Your body isn't everything. It's not the whole of who you are. It's a container. That is not to say that it's not important to keep it healthy and strong so that you can live a long and healthy life; but dieting, starving and bingeing isn't healthy. Your body is a safe. It needs to be strong only because it holds all the good stuff. Your body is disposable. The good stuff – the warmth, the compassion, the love, the intelligence, the creativity, the kindness and everything else – stays secure inside of it. It's just a body. Weight is just a number on a scale, calories are just a unit of heat, size is just the measure of matter. The meaning that we attach to it has no bearing on who you are as a person. It doesn't measure your heart, your intelligence, your insight, your warmth; it just measures how much physical space you take up. That's it. Nothing else. Weight is a fact, not a moral judgment, yet we seem to attach so much more to it.

People often talk about a "goal weight". What is a "goal weight"? It's an arbitrary number that's not grounded in reality. Who tells you what your goal weight should be? How is that realistic?

If you are a normal weight, and your body holds onto it, despite what you do to it, you have to know that this is a healthy response from a healthy body. You are blessed. A healthy body wants to maintain the homeostasis. You can run millions of miles, you can binge, you can starve, you can purge, you can diet, you can use laxatives, but no matter how much you abuse your body, if you are healthy, and your body wants to stay healthy, it will fight. It will do what it can to maintain the homeostasis. Of course you can push it too far and make yourself sick. But often, if you are putting lots and lots and lots of exhausting effort into losing weight and your body won't budge, you probably have a healthy body that is trying to stay that way.

Rather than a goal weight, your goal should be health. Your goal should be a long healthy life with love, with adventure, with fun, with pain, with sorrow, with self-love, with self-criticism, with anger, with sadness, with joy, with excitement, with ups, with downs. But your goals should have nothing to do with sizes and numbers.

Even if you are not at a weight that is healthy for you, if you are generally healthy, your body will do what it can to get to its healthy number, and that might have nothing to do with what the BMI says, or with what Hollywood says or with what the MetLife height and weight chart says. When your body is healthy, it knows where it should go. Treat it with love and respect. Feed it, exercise it, water it. Give it lots of fruit, lots of veggies, lots of protein, and even let it have a piece of cake or slice of pizza or a glass of wine every now and again. When you set yourself free from the obsession of a number, your body has the freedom to comfortably fall to its right size.

Those who find themselves obsessed with their weight are often avoiding something much bigger. That doesn't include just those who fixate on their own weights, but those who fixate on others' weights and body sizes as well. Many women believe that potential partners are only interested in thin women. Some men and women are and some are not. However, in choosing a partner, it's of dire importance to choose someone who sees all of you, not just your outward appearance, which fades as soon as a person opens her mouth and lets out what's really inside.

Miranda, a 21-year-old art student, had an obsession with being thin. However, as an artist and a nonconformist, she claimed that she was someone who valued intellect, compassion, kindness, artistic prowess and originality over conforming to society's rigid view on appearance and the significant value it placed on thinness. Yet, despite the fact that Miranda claimed she was appalled by popular culture's emphasis on keeping the female body small, she was very caught up in the tyranny of thinness. She said that she thought that it was okay for other women to be curvy or voluptuous and even admired a body like that on others; yet for her, it was not okay. During one of our sessions, she explained to me that having a skinny body was important because it would let people know who she was. Miranda struggled with crippling social anxiety. Speaking to people elicited so much anxiety that she found herself rarely answering people's questions, or shrugging her shoulders when she was spoken to. She didn't want to be that way; however, she couldn't find words and feared that what she said would not be well received. She explained to me that staying skinny would control what people's perception of her was. She believed that if she were thin, she wouldn't have to talk or have a personality because they would already know what kind of person she was, an in-control person, a person of substance and moral fiber, someone who was secure and who had her shit together.

"People will get all this just from looking at you and seeing that you are thin?"

"Yes," she told me.

Rather than working on dealing with her social anxiety and her insecurity, it was easier for Miranda to fixate on being thin. She believed that it would solve all her problems. The truth was, Miranda was quite thin. She was also quite bulimic. She would binge and purge several times each day in her quest to convince people that she was well. Of course she was quite unwell.

"What does it matter how sick I am as long as people think that I'm perfect?" she asked me.

"Well," I said, "I'll ask you the converse question. Does it

237

mean anything if people think you are perfect, yet you are so sick?"

"How can I think that I'm great if no one else does?"

"How can anyone else think that you're great when you don't? You don't know what other people are thinking. You don't have to live with anyone else's thoughts, just your own."

This is common, this scenario and this attitude. I've heard this from clients over and over. Is it familiar to you? One thing that an Eating Disorder tricks us into believing is that we have control over people's thoughts and perceptions of us. That is completely untrue. The only thoughts that we have control over are our own. You can be the most perfect, most selfless, most beautiful, most thin, most self-sacrificing person in the world, and still, there will be people who hate you. That's why no American President has ever had a 100% approval rating. That's why there are documentaries and exposés about Mother Teresa.

As I said earlier, the unavoidable result of trying to be perfect all the time is an extremely low self-esteem. Another one of my 'perfect patients' was Brenda, a 25-year-old woman with a perfect boyfriend, a perfect apartment, a perfect body, perfect clothes, perfect skin, and perfect hair. However, she had a raging case of bulimia nervosa. We discussed her outward self and how she presented a façade of perfection; and how it didn't serve her at all. She was very angry when I suggested that she become more open and honest with people about who she really was and what she was really thinking. It was never okay for her to be emotional or sloppy in front of people. If she ever made a mistake, she was absolutely mortified. Suggesting that she allow some room for being human left her with a bad taste in her mouth. "Being perfect is serving me," she told me. "My life is pretty great the way it is; everyone loves me, I have tons of friends, everyone thinks I'm awesome," she told me.

"Yes," I told her, "everyone loves you except for you, because you go home, make yourself vomit every single night. How is that your life going great?"

"What does it matter?" she asked me. "Only you and me know about that; everyone else sees me as totally put together, everyone thinks I have it all."

"Does it matter how others see you if you, the only person who has to live with yourself, the only person who really truly knows yourself, believe that you are so flawed?"

Bulimia is the ultimate manifestation of all or nothing thinking. Bulimia is the anthropomorphosis of black and white thinking. All the food in, you are full; all the food out and you are empty.

You have to work on liking yourself. Your body is your outward appearance. It's your container; it holds all the good stuff. It should be kept healthy for your own sense of self-worth and well-being. Healthy is eating right, exercising regularly and sending loving thoughts to your body.

Common Comments and My Answers

1. Why should I love my body when it's so fat?
The only way to change is through self-acceptance. How can you lovingly care for something that you hate? The more you hate your body, the more you punish it with strict dieting, bingeing, purging, laxative use, compulsive exercise, drugs, alcohol, and other things. The more you love it, the more you are likely to respect it and treat it well. When you treat it well, your body will come to a weight that is right for you. Your body doesn't want to be painfully thin; your body doesn't want to be obese either. When you love and nurture it, it will naturally come to a place that is pleasing to you.

2. I will definitely stop dieting and start loving my body as soon as these last 10 pounds are gone.
You can't wait. You've waited long enough already. How long

have you been trying to lose those pounds? How long has your life been on hold as you scheme the next diet, the next exercise regimen, the next dress size that you are going to fit into. Life isn't about trying to fit into a certain size for a certain event. Life is about living. If you wait, you will miss it.

3. Everyone else seems to be able to stay thin without dieting, but in my case, it just isn't true.

This is the compare-despair trap; you compare yourself to others and then you feel horrible. It is a trap because you are caught up in the stories that you are creating in your own mind. You have absolutely no idea what is going on in other people's minds or what their behaviors are behind closed doors. Life is challenging for everyone because we are all born into a series of challenges and tests and strength-building exercises. Even though it is so difficult, you can try to accept that you have these challenges and that it is your dharma or your path to persevere and work through them in order to continue with and shape your life.

4. Does it mean that I'm a bad person just because I want to be thinner?

Wanting to be thinner definitely does not make you superficial or self-absorbed or shallow or a bad person. However, when you focus all your energy on wanting to be thin, you begin to neglect the other parts of you that are important. You begin constantly perusing the Internet for the next best diet plan, you obsess on what the number on the scale says, you become consumed with how many calories or grams of fat there are in the food that you eat. With all this obsessing, you come to completely neglect yourself and your life. You forget who you really are and get caught up in the belief that you won't be valid or worthy until you are that number. You become your diet – it plagues you and stops you from living your life. When you begin to pay attention to who you are and nurture your own talents, skills, passions, do the things that you love and become engaged in your life, you will find that your fixation on food and calories decreases. As it decreases, you begin to feel satisfied with who you are and find comfort in your being as you become an active participant in your life rather than someone waiting to join it. You are more than just an arbitrary number on a scale that might never come.

5. If I let myself like my body, it will become fatter; I will become so obese that I won't be able to live with myself. Calling it names and being mean to it is the way that I keep myself in line.
Something is wrong here. Would you teach a child to read by calling him or her stupid every time they made a mistake? Would you beat a child every time they had an accident while learning to potty train? If you did, what would happen? This child would be so afraid of making a mistake that he or she would shut down and be unable to learn. They would believe that they were worthless, stupid and unable, and they would continue to make in their pants and believe that they could never learn to read. It is the same thing with your body. If you constantly berate yourself, you will begin to truly believe that there is something very wrong with you. You will find that you are violently restricting and withholding food from yourself one day, then bingeing on those same foods the next. You will hold the belief that you are a failure and worthless. As important as it is to be kind to people around you, it's important to be kind to your body.

Exercise One: Body Gratitude – *Journal Opportunity*
This exercise is about showing gratitude to each part of your body for carrying you through your lifetime. For each body part, write down what you feel thankful for; then look toward it, and as you read the sentiment out loud, touch that part of your body with love and respect.

Thank you, toes, for:

Thank you, ankles, for:

Thank you, calves, for:

Thank you, knees, for:

Thank you, thighs, for:

Thank you, hips, for:

Thank you, belly, for:

Thank you, chest, for:

Thank you, arms, for:

Thank you, hands, for:

Thank you, face, for:

Thank you, nose, for:

Thank you, eyes, for:

Thank you, ears, for:

Thank you, head, for:

Thank you, body, for:

Exercise Two: Letter Writing

Write a Hate Letter to the body part that you hate the most:

Now, write a response to yourself from that body part:

Write a note of apology for all that you've said, done and put your body through:

Write a love letter to the part of your body that you dislike the most:

Exercise Three: Understanding the Impact of Body Acceptance

1. If I had to give up dieting, the thing about myself that I'd have to focus on would be:

2. It would be hard for me to focus on this because:

3. If I didn't have food or bingeing to give me comfort and solace, I am afraid that:

4. If I decided to accept my body as it is, the negative outcome of this would be:

5. If I decided to accept my body as it is, the positive outcome of this would be:

Step Twenty-Six – Body Trust: Learning to Listen to the Wisdom of Your Body

When you were born, you intuitively knew how much food you needed. You knew when to ask for food and you knew when you were ready to stop eating. This probably was not always respected as your caregivers might have wanted you to eat "just one more bite… please" and as you got older, people might have commented on how small you were or how big you were. Then, as you became more cognizant of your body and you began to take note of people making comments that you'd put on some weight or that you were getting fat or other comments on your body, you began to second-guess what you were eating.

Patrice, a 42-year-old homemaker, had actually been on a very low carbohydrate diet for over 31 years. Patrice didn't know that she was fat at the time that her mother first started her on it. In fact, when she brought in pictures to share from that time in her life, she appeared to be an average, healthy pre-teen. Patrice's mom felt the need to 'nip it in the bud' before it became a problem. Of course, it became a problem. Patrice was taught by her mother not to trust her appetite. She began to restrict Patrice's food and track her eating meticulously. The message that Patrice learned was that she could not trust herself to eat what she wanted to; that it would make her fat. She began to put all her faith in the plan and avoid her own needs for food. She would go weeks eating nothing but steak and broccoli, then binge on the cookies and cakes that her friends were eating at birthday parties. Where her friends would only have one piece of cake or a few cookies, Patrice knew that this was her one opportunity until the tyranny of her mother's strict diet. She would try to get every last bit in while she could, then return to celery sticks and seltzer at home. As Patrice became an adult, her mother's iron fist was transferred into her and she became the one who ruled over herself so ruthlessly. It was she who would deprive herself of treats and then, when her faculties were low, that part of her who would binge on treats when her mom wasn't around, that part would take over. When the iron fist came back, Patrice would punish herself; go back to steak and broccoli. Ironically, with all that bingeing and dieting and all those years, Patrice never really deviated from one weight. She was either five pounds above it or five pounds below it.

In recovery, Patrice first had to give up the notion of dieting. As you can imagine, this was challenging for her. She relied on her plan to give her structure. She relied on her weekly weigh-ins to keep her in line. It was her religion. However, she contended that she was not actually living. She was avoiding life by letting the plan be her life. It took her almost two years to actually give up dieting. She would try for a few days, and then be too afraid to trust her own needs.

She started off slowly; at first she would just not count carbs on one meal. Then, she would take a day and not count carbs. Then, she would go a whole week. In the beginning, it was challenging and she found that not counting turned into a binge. However, as she began to realize that she was allowed to have another meal that would be unrestricted, she was able to make better choices. She knew that she didn't have to eat until she was uncomfortably full, because she was allowed to have what she wanted at each meal. As she became mindful both in therapy and with her body, she began to be able to feed it what she needed.

Being mindful in therapy meant being honest about what she was feeling and not avoiding the truly painful things. This enabled her to listen to her body more completely. The control that Patrice's mother exerted over her daughter's food trans-formed into Patrice needing to have power and control over her own feelings. By allowing herself to be with the real scary and uncomfortable feelings in therapy, she was able to be more mindful about what she was feeling in her body. Our therapy sessions were hard; there was a lot that she hadn't been openly acknowledging. She was unhappy in her marriage; she felt that she gave up on her career to marry and have children. But as we began to acknowledge that, there was actually a way that she could change that. She started taking some classes and reintroduced into her life yoga and sculpture, two things that she'd been passionate about before marriage and kids. She and her husband entered couples counseling so that they could really talk about what was going on. Patrice's life was becoming fuller. She was more integrated into her body, and so she was able to understand what she was feeling both physically and emotionally.

Before she ate, Patrice would close her eyes, tune in to her body and ask what it needed. Sometimes it said that it needed greens, sometimes it needed red meat and other times it needed fruit. There were other times that her body would tell her that it needed to eat a whole cake by herself. She was able to know that her body did not necessarily need to eat a whole cake. She would look for other feelings that she might have been having. If no feelings came up for her, or she was unable to identify what she was feeling, she'd settle on a healthy meal and allow herself one piece of cake for dessert. This was usually sufficient and she didn't suffer with the level of guilt that she had in the past for eating off plan. In allowing herself to tune in to her body, she began to trust that it would lead her to what it needed. Her weight stabilized; she was no longer five pounds up or five pounds down, she came to a place that she felt comfortable at. When her mother came to visit and saw her eating a croissant at breakfast, she said, "Oh my God, don't you know how many carbohydrates are in that?" She simply replied, "Nope. And I don't care to know." She felt that she had learned the real secret to body trust. Nurture your body by giving it what it needs when it needs it, and it's okay to have a little something extra – that you can enjoy in a healthy, moderate way at times. Your body knows how to find its right size.

Meditation Time

At least an hour before each meal, close your eyes and be silent. Begin to let your breath lead you. Watch your breath and allow your thoughts to be whatever they may, but try not to follow them; don't engage with them. Just come back to your breath. When you are feeling calm, ask your body what it needs and be silent. As you listen to the silence, you will receive an answer.

Exercise: The Mindful Meal – The Next Level

Give yourself several hours for this mindful meal. The mindful meal actually begins with the mindful grocery-shopping excursion.

Begin by sitting down at the table and asking your body what it needs. Be silent and listen. It might tell you that it needs green vegetables, or red meat, or fruit, or whole grains, or fat. Try to 'hear' intuitively what your body needs. As you do, make a shopping list and find or create a recipe for the foods that you chose. When you go to the store, don't deviate from the list. Just buy what you've set out to. Take your time at the supermarket. Notice the sights, notice the people in the market. Do some people seem like they are mindlessly dropping things in their carts, hypnotized by food and oblivious to their surroundings? Do some people stick rigidly to lists, reading labels obsessively? Do some people seem lost and confused? Do some people seem happy, alive and in their bodies? Are there children? What are they doing? What are their reactions to food? What are their parents' reactions to them? Watch and just take note of what you see. Next, take note of what you feel. Are you being triggered by certain aisles? Is the noise or are the crowds making you want to buy all the food you can and run away to binge alone? Are you feeling as though you want to eat because of the visual stimulation of all that food? Are you hungry? Notice how you feel as you fill your cart. Notice what your body does. Does your stomach growl? Does your mouth water as you see certain foods? Are you feeling anxious or excited just being in the store? There's no need to do anything or judge what you're feeling, just take note. If you have your journal with you, you might write some quick notes about what you notice. Choose the foods that are on your list. Do you find that you want to buy things that are not on your list? Take note of that, but just for today choose not to give in to that urge. Today you are just letting yourself notice your thoughts and feelings without judging them or acting on them. Who you are and what you feel is valid and important. People often tell me that they have all these feelings and they don't know what to do with them. The answer is, there is nothing to do with them. Just allow them to be and give them validation and acknowledgement.

After you pay for your food, notice your trip home. Are you anxious to eat? Excited to prepare a meal for yourself? Dreading it? Again, just note what you're feeling. When you get home, allow yourself to prepare your meal with care. If you are cutting your vegetables, feel what it's like to slice, be aware of the sensations in your fingers, in your hands. Notice your instincts. Do you want to get this done quickly or are you enjoying the process? Slow down and try to allow yourself to be with the process. Try not to speed up just to get things done. When you are finally ready to eat, make sure that there is no music on, no television, no Internet, no other people, just you and your food. When you eat, look at your food. Chew it slowly. Notice what it is like to savor your food. Notice the tastes. Notice the sensations of chewing. Notice the sensation of swallowing. Notice how your digestion process feels. Notice your emotions. One patient of mine was very aware that she was filled with anger and rage while doing a mindful meal. She realized that she had been stuffing food quickly in order to quell her rage. Mindful meals were very difficult for her because she was very uncomfortable with that rage. However, as she learned to contact that rage and be with it in therapy sessions and outside, she found that she wasn't eating as furiously and quickly as she had been.

As you eat your meal, continue to check in with your body to see if you need more food, or if you're beginning to feel satisfied. Try to stop eating when you feel satisfied, but before you feel full. What does that feel like? Do you have the urge to eat until you are stuffed? Is it challenging to stop eating when you are satisfied, or is it easy? When you are finished with your meal, either call someone to talk about your experience or write about it. Notice what you feel like. Are you satisfied? Satiated? Do you have the urge to binge? Are you still hungry? Are you full? What thoughts and feelings are emerging?

When you begin to trust the wisdom of your body, peace around food can be yours.

Step Twenty-Seven –
Dealing with Saboteurs

When you begin taking care of yourself, you might notice that people around you, friends and family members might become angry and even try to sabotage your growth and healing. This is not because close friends and relatives want to hurt you. This is because as human beings, we will do anything to maintain the homeostasis. We are used to what we know, and we don't like change. Every time something changes within a system, every part of the system is forced to change along with it, thus we will fight against change.

This is the big irony of recovery: the people around us want us to change, but when we do, they begin to feel threatened. Why? Because when you change, it forces the people around you to change as well. For instance, if you have spent years stuffing your feelings, and now, as you work through your recovery, you begin to speak up for your needs, set boundaries, and voice your resentments, the people you are closest to might feel very uncomfortable with that. They might not know how to react and thus be very unsupportive of your needs. Another example is that you might have someone who you used to binge eat or compulsively diet with, a friend or even a partner. When you choose to let go of these behaviors, your partner in diet crime might feel left behind. However, it is not your responsibility to engage them in your new healthy habits, or encourage them to start their own healthy regimens. It is also not your fault if they are unhappy with your recovery program. You have to take care of your needs and trust those around you to take care of their own needs or to learn how to take care of their needs. If you don't choose yourself first then who will? Everyone is given a body and a soul, and we each have the responsibility of taking care of that body and soul. If we reject ourselves to take care of someone else (besides our children), we not only hurt ourselves, we also take away the opportunity for our loved ones to learn to take care of themselves. It will be tempting to sacrifice your own wants and needs for others, but you have to remember that this won't benefit anyone in the long-term. It may help you to avoid conflict in the present moment, but as you continue to sacrifice yourself for others, resentment grows inside until you eventually spill over. Tristan, a 28-year-old patient of mine, found that when she spent time with her sister, she would always wind up binge eating. They would go to a certain Mexican restaurant that they had always enjoyed together and wind up eating food and drinking margaritas until they were uncomfortably full. Tristan admitted that it felt impossible for her to tell her sister that she couldn't go to that restaurant. She didn't want to upset her sister; she didn't want her sister to feel abandoned or as though there was something wrong with her because she wasn't actively in recovery. Tristan was also protective of her own fragile recovery and feared that it would be vulnerable to criticism if she told her sister about it. She and her sister were both victims of extreme child abuse. The way they took care of themselves and each other growing up was by binge eating together. This was an experience that both bonded them and helped them numb out the pain of severe physical and sexual abuse. Because of this, Tristan felt that not bingeing with her sister would be a betrayal. She would be betraying her sister the way their dad had betrayed them. Of course this was not conscious at first, but as she began to untangle some of the issues around food and binge eating and family, it became apparent.

Some friends or family might accuse you of "not being a team player" if you refuse to eat with them the way you used to. Some people might feel uncomfortable with your new eating habits or your weight loss because it changes their position. People are comfortable with who you are and who they are in relation to you. When you begin to change, it forces them to change. The change is challenging not just for you, but for the people around you. Don't underestimate the effect that one person's behavior has on the people around them, even behaviors toward oneself. As a binge eater, you assume a certain role. You might be the one in your family who holds all the emotions, the one who is there for everyone. You might be the funny one, the one who brings levity to all situations. You might be the fat one. You might be the one who takes care of everyone and avoids her needs. Whatever it is that you are, when you begin to focus on healing yourself, you change your position in the family. You will begin to create boundaries. You will first begin by creating boundaries with food, but then, you will begin to create boundaries with people around you. You will start saying no when people ask you for favors that you just can't commit to. You will begin to let people solve their own problems. You will refuse to engage in unhealthy eating behaviors with other people.

These changes won't just be challenging for you, they will be for anyone around you. There will be a grieving period when you let go of your old ways of being. As you go through the stages of grief you will find that the people around you are going through their own grieving process as they don't want to let go of the 'old' you.

For you, the grieving process might look like this:

Denial: I don't need to do anything different. My issues with binge eating have nothing to do with anything other than willpower. I just have to stop eating and I'll be fine. Once I lose the weight, my life will be better.

Anger: This is ridiculous. Life seems really hard all of a sudden. I have all these uncomfortable feelings. I don't know why I had to stir up all of these emotions. There was no reason to do it. I hate this. Bingeing is better than sitting with these emotions.

Bargaining: I think that I can reasonably go back on the diet that's worked before, and lose the weight without having to go through all of this recovery stuff. If I just start now, I'll lose the weight and everything will be fine.

Depression: This is never going to be better. I'm always going to be stuck with this.

Acceptance: What I've been doing for all these years, dieting and bingeing and eating my emotions, hasn't worked so I'm going to let go and surrender to my recovery and take care of myself emotionally in a way that I haven't done before. It will be challenging, but in the long run, my life will be better for it.

For people around you, the grieving process might look like this:

Denial: Great! She's starting another diet again. I'm sure that it will fail miserably the way all of her diets do. Whatever, there's no reason for me to be scared; nothing is going to change. She'll be eating nachos with me the second I see her.

Anger: What's wrong with her? When I asked her to do me this favor, she refused. That's not fair; she has always done the things that I've asked her to do. But now that she's in recovery she's trying to take care of herself? That feels really bad. Where am I? Why is she neglecting me? If she is taking care of herself, then who will take care of me?

Bargaining: Maybe I'll take her out to dinner to a meal that I know she usually binges on. I know that she won't be able to refuse and then things will be the way they used to.

Depression: Things will never be the same. I lost my best friend. I'm alone and lonely and I have no idea who I am.

Acceptance: Just because she's taking care of herself doesn't mean that I can't take care of myself. If she's really my friend, I will feel happy for her, not threatened and jealous. I understand that it has been a hard transition and change for me, but as I support her in her recovery, I can also support myself in being more independent. Without food and favors and resentment between us, our friendship can be more pure and deeper.

Unfortunately, you might lose some friends in the process of recovery. Those are the friends who were so invested in you being sick because it gave them a sense of who they were or even made them feel better about themselves. They are unable to accept that you are getting better. Those friends who you lose deserve some compassion because they might not feel very good about themselves. They might be uncomfortable in their own skin and need you to be sick to feel better about themselves rather than working from within to take care of themselves. Though you can feel compassion, you do not need to take care of them. That's an inside job.

Exercise One: Identifying Your Saboteurs – *Journal Opportunity*

1. Is there anyone in your life with whom you binge eat or use food with in a ritualized way? If so, who?
2. How does this serve or enhance your relationship?
3. What are your fears about telling this person that you no longer want food to be the center of your friendship?
4. What other things might you do that can serve a similar purpose as food did?
5. Can you present this to your friend in a compassionate way? If so, how?

Exercise Two: Identifying Systems that Perpetuate Your Binge Eating – *Journal Opportunity*

1. Is there anyone who would be threatened by your recovery? Who?

2. What do you think would be threatening?
3. How can you handle it with compassion if this person tries to sabotage your recovery?
4. How will you take care of yourself if people become angry about you beginning to prioritize yourself and your recovery?

Exercise Three: Creating Boundaries – *Journal Opportunity*

1. Your best friend has had a horrible day. She found out that her boyfriend has been cheating on her, she got laid off, and to top it off, her mother is in the hospital. She calls you up in tears and wants you to come over for pizza and brownies and ice cream and movies. How do you handle this compassionately while still taking care of yourself?

2. It's a Friday night and you have nothing planned. It's been a long week and you just want to stay home and take a bubble bath and relax. Your brother calls you and asks if you can come over and babysit. He and your sister-in-law would really like a much needed date night and know that you have no plans that night. How do you create boundaries and handle this compassionately while still taking care of yourself?

3. You are having dinner with your family and your mom brings out a big dessert that has always been a giant trigger food for you. You know that if you start in on it, you will probably spend the night (and maybe even the next several days) bingeing. She knows that you've been working on recovery from binge eating and food issues. How do you gently but firmly remind her that this isn't okay and she needs to be supportive?

4. And what if she acts insulted or has hurt feelings?
5. It's your birthday and your girlfriends surprise you by

bringing you to one of your old favorite haunts, which, incidentally, is a place that has triggered binges in the past. How do you handle this situation with grace while still taking care of yourself?

6. You are beginning to recover and take better care of yourself, learning to say no to people, and learning how to create boundaries around food, when one of your close friends tells you that you're changing for the worse and she doesn't know that she can be your friend anymore. How do you feel about this? And how do you deal with this?

Dealing with People's Comments

Something that many of my patients deal with is having people around them comment on what they are eating and how they are eating. Remember that you don't owe anyone an explanation about what you choose to eat or not to eat. People are naturally curious about other people's food:

"What are you eating there?"
"Really, you don't eat that?"
"Wow, you can really eat a lot!"
"Seriously, that's all you're eating?"
"I never see you eating, when do you ever eat?"

These are common and often innocent comments and questions. For someone with an eating disorder, though, these are invasive, off-putting and can feel very intrusive. You might feel as though your boundaries are being completely violated. There is absolutely no reason to justify your choices to anyone. You can answer with something as obtuse as, "I'm just not that hungry today" or "I'm just not eating it right now" or "Yes, I can eat a lot." Or you can turn around, not answer the question and ask the person the same question. That will often send the hint that this is a subject that's not up for discussion. Example:

"You barely eat!"

– Of course I eat.

"Why don't you eat lunch?"

– I eat lunch.

"I never see you."

– Why? Are you trying to find me eating lunch?

"I thought you were a vegetarian!"

– Sometimes I eat vegetarian, sometimes I don't.

"I thought you were allergic to wheat! You said that two weeks ago!"

– I thought I was too. But, apparently not.

Monica, a 23-year-old patient of mine, came in with severe food obsession. She'd tried everything from no sugar, to no fat, to no wheat, to no dairy, to no yeast, to all fruit, to all fish. Each time she got on a new bandwagon, she made a grandiose statement to everyone she worked with about how she was 'gluten sensitive', or 'insulin resistant' or a whole plethora of other food-based maladies that she believed she might be victim to. As she began to recover and let go of her restrictions, she found a new problem, which was that she was being 'inspected' at work. People kept on asking her why she was eating this or that when she previously said that she couldn't. It was so overwhelming to her that she began to eat her lunch in a stall in a bathroom.

As we worked together, she realized that she couldn't allow other people's intrusiveness to rule her life or her eating. She realized that she had to learn to create boundaries with people. She began to tell people that actually she found that she was feeling fine. That she was integrating more foods and was feeling healthier than ever. Eventually people got tired of asking and let her alone to eat what she chose to eat.

Step Twenty-Eight – Feeling Jealous, Envious and Making Comparisons

"Other people don't have the same problems that I have."

"All of my friends are tall and thin and beautiful and in relationships; they don't have issues with food. They eat when they are hungry and stop when they are satisfied."

"She is so much better than me. She's smarter, more successful, prettier, has a better relationship, has more money, is thinner, dresses better… she has it all and I have nothing."

"That woman at the bar drinking the martini can have any man she wants. Every guy in here is staring at her and not one person is paying any attention to me at all…"

"Everyone has a husband or a boyfriend or a significant other, yet I can't even get a date…"

"Everyone around me has a baby, yet I can't get pregnant."

Many women have the habit of comparing their lives to the lives of someone else and then feeling bad about themselves. Compare and Despair. Or, as one of my former supervisors referred to it, "Compare and Destroy". When you compare yourself to other people, you can often wind up obliterating yourself or the other person. Often, people believe that making comparisons, measuring yourself against another person, can be a way of understanding where you fall, how you're doing. We don't get graded in life. So, perhaps if we can see who has the most money, the thinnest legs, the biggest house, the handsomest husband, we can understand where we stand.

This can be particularly true with body image. Many women spend a good part of their day and their mind space comparing their bodies to the bodies of other women and then feeling badly about themselves. This kind of comparison is so detrimental to your mental and emotional health. It pulls you away from you. You become so busy looking at what other people have that you begin to forget about yourself. This isn't only true about comparing yourself to a body that you think is 'better' than yours, it's also when you compare yourself to a body that you think is 'worse' than yours. There are no qualitative parameters on bodies. You have only been given one body and it is your responsibility alone to care for it. Each person has their own dharma and their own path. It's up to you to travel along on your own path, to go forward and figure out all your obstacles and roadblocks. When you compare yourself to others, you begin to look to other people's paths. In doing that, you stop moving forward on your own. You can't jump on anyone else's path. You have your own. Each person has their own life and their own problems. When you compare yourself and your life to other people, you are not taking into consideration that you don't actually know what's going on in their lives. You are comparing yourself to a fantasy that you are having about someone else's life.

Sonia, a 36-year-old woman, used to come in to see me every Tuesday at 5pm. Sonia was dealing with compulsive eating and relationship issues and believed that the extra 20 pounds that she was holding was the reason that she could not find a boyfriend. One day, she came in and told me that she needed to change her time. "I can't stand that woman you see before me," she told me. "Just looking at her turns my stomach; it brings up all of my feelings of inadequacy."

"What does that mean?" I asked her.

"Well first off, she's got that giant diamond ring on her finger. She can't be over 30 and she's happily married to apparently a very rich guy. Secondly, she's gorgeous and thin, and clearly has tons of money based on that ring and her big designer purse. She's always dressed to the nines and I'm just totally jealous. Just looking at her upsets me. I feel totally like shit about myself."

The patient who came in before Sonia was under 30, and was married to a very rich man and was very beautiful. But she also suffered from a crippling case of Crohn's disease. Her flare-ups were intense and she spent a significant amount of time in bed and not being out in the world. She was a professional dancer and had been in the Ballet; but due to her illness, her career was coming to an end and her marriage was suffering greatly. Although her husband was loving and kind, he had a lot of trouble dealing with his own feelings about her illness and wound up drinking and dabbling in some extramarital affairs.

What is so ironic here is that Sonia had her whole life ahead of her. But she was a slave to her own mind. She was comparing herself to someone who was a slave to her illness and trapped in a body that was attacking and destroying itself. Sonia couldn't have known this. But she looked outside of herself and escaped into fantasies about other people in order to compare and then destroy herself. You have to look at what you have and work with that. That is all you can do. Expending energy on being envious brings you away from what you want for yourself, and also wastes so much time and mind space.

I worked with a patient who said that when she noticed she was doing that, she would try to "bring it back in". Comparing herself to others and feeling the pain of being angry at what she didn't have really pulled her away from herself and kept her vulnerable to binge eating and binge drinking as well. If she noticed that she was engaging in comparative thinking, she'd say the word "Stop" out loud. Then she would pull herself out of it and think about what she needed. Then, she would do the next right thing. The next right thing is anything healthy that you can do to take care of yourself. This can be stocking your kitchen with healthy foods, going to the gym, flossing your teeth, calling your grandma... whatever is your next right thing.

Exercise: Dealing with Jealousy – *Journal Opportunity*

1.   Are there any people who you are jealous or envious of?

Who?

2. What do they have that you want?
3. How do you know that you want that?
4. How would your life be different if you had that?
5. How do you know that is true?
6. What's good and exciting about your own life?
7. What have you learned from your own struggles?
8. Are there people in the world who you had thought in the past had it all, but then learned that they had their own crosses to bear? If so, who and what was the situation?
9. When you notice yourself comparing yourself to someone else, what are some ways that you can stop yourself?
10. How can you "bring it back in" when you are engaging in comparative thinking?

Step Twenty-Nine – Exercise

Of course you know that exercise is super important for health. It is great for cardiovascular health, and it greatly reduces symptoms of anxiety and depression. It's also associated with improved cognition and memory as well as preventing and controlling diabetes, lowering blood pressure, reducing your risk of stroke, decreasing your risk of osteoporosis and helping you to sleep longer and better.

If you haven't been a regular exerciser, you will find that implementing a regular exercise program increases feelings of calmness and well-being while decreasing symptoms of anxiety and stress. You don't have to start by joining a gym and spending an hour on the treadmill each day. Exercise can be as simple as putting your iPod on and taking a walk through your neighborhood. It can be doing a yoga video in your living room. If you find that you are unable to motivate yourself to start an exercise regimen, enlist a friend or a few friends to go on walks or runs, or go to classes or do videos a few times a week. Make it enjoyable and have tangible goals for yourself. Rather than, "I'll go to the gym every day this week," have something in mind like, "I will move for 30 minutes four days this week."

However, just like with food, it is possible to be incredibly unhealthy with exercise. When it comes to exercise, too much of a good thing can turn into a very bad thing.

Usually, compulsive exercise manifests as the need to exercise every day no matter what. Irene, a very high functioning 28-year-old investment banker, had to run ten miles every day no matter what. She got into work each morning at 7am, but was up at 4am each morning to do her run, no matter how tired she was, no matter whether or not she was sick, or even injured. If for some reason she had to skip a run in the morning, she would find a way to either squeeze one in during the day or in the evening.

The idea of not running in the morning was incredibly panic inducing for her. She had this belief that if she stopped running every single morning, she would get very fat. At this point, exercise goes from being something healthy to something compulsive. Rather than enhancing your health, it destroys your health.

Though it's true that many people feel defeated about the fact that they cannot get themselves to exercise, several of my patients tend to do the opposite and binge on exercise. Exercise can be incredibly compulsive and unhealthy. Many people have a picture in their minds of compulsive exercisers being super thin and fit. However, that's simply not always the case. Compulsive exercisers come in all shapes and sizes, from very small to quite large.

Compulsive exercise can also be called exercise bulimia, because people try to compensate for the food that they've eaten by burning it off with exercise. Sally, a 30-year-old grad student, used to try to calculate the amount of calories that she'd eaten in a binge, and then spend hours at the gym on the elliptical trainer trying to burn them off. There was even one day that she spent almost nine hours on the elliptical machine trying to compensate for eating a whole pizza pie and a gallon of ice cream she'd consumed. She got to the gym early in the morning after staying up all night bingeing and didn't leave until after 2pm. The only reason she left was because she was asked to by the facility. This was incredibly embarrassing and traumatizing for Sally, because she was noticed and called out in her disorder by other people. She never went into that gym again, but she did begin to notice that she had a very big problem. Exercise had taken over her life. She would skip classes to exercise, she would skip social engagements, and if for some reason she was completely unable to exercise, she would compensate by either purging or not eating at all that day. On that particular day, she even skipped the midterm that she'd been up all night studying for and bingeing over. The interesting thing to note about Sally is that she was a woman of size. No matter how much and how intensely she exercised, her body shape did not dramatically shift. This is an extreme case of exercise bulimia. Because her case was so extreme, I put her on complete exercise restriction. She had to cut out all exercise for three months. This felt impossible to her and she certainly found that she was not able to restrict her exercise on many days. However, on the days that she didn't exercise, she found that she was incredibly distressed, anxious, sad, lonely and angry. She began to realize that she wasn't exercising in a healthy way, but using exercise to run away from her feelings. She'd sustained several injuries from the excessive exercise, and coupled with her bingeing, purging and restricting she had put undue strain on her heart. Her compulsive exercise was putting her life at risk, but she found that she wasn't able to stop because the feelings that ensued on the days that she didn't exercise were totally overwhelming. She insisted that the emotions that came up for her on the days that she did not exercise were fear of getting fat; but as we continued working together, she did come to see that the need to change her body and the obsession with that need helped her to block out every other thing going on in her life.

Eventually, she learned to exercise moderately and in a way that was healthy. She even integrated gentle yoga into her exercise regimen a few times a week. She never got skinny the way she thought 'should' be, her body had other ideas; but she found that as she evened out into moderate exercise and moderate eating, her weight began to stabilize to a place that she eventually made peace with.

But What About Professional Athletes?

It is true that professional athletes do train more vigorously and intensely than most people. Of course professional athletes have to deal with the constant threat of injury destroying their livelihood. Unlike compulsive exercisers, their whole job is to train, so they are not trying to balance training with another full-time job. They also have nutritionists, teams of sports doctors, physical therapists, and they get paid to train. Their careers have a shelf life though, and many still wind up with a plethora of injuries and maladies from overtraining.

How Do You Know if You're a Compulsive Exerciser?

How do you know when exercise is compulsive rather than just healthy?

Ask yourself these questions:

1. Do you get upset or anxious if you can't exercise every single day?
2. Do you forgo social invitations in order to exercise?
3. Do you make sure that you always exercise on vacations or trips away?
4. Do you exercise when you're sick or injured?
5. Do you exercise past the point of exhaustion, to where you feel like you just can't go anymore, but you continue to?
6. Do you use exercise to compensate for the amount that you've eaten? For instance, do you count the calories that you've eaten, and then try to exercise off the same amount of calories?
7. Do you have overtraining syndrome? Symptoms include:
Getting sick often
Night Sweats
Insomnia
Fatigue
Chronic Soreness and Joint Inflammation
Injuries
Headaches
Waking up too early

If you are someone who puts exercise ahead of the rest of your life, and you said yes to one of these, you might be compulsive with exercise; and if you said yes to more than one, there's a very high probability that you are a compulsive exerciser. As with any eating disorder, compulsive exercise can be extremely dangerous. There is the possibility of severe injury or heart attack if you completely ignore your bodily cues and sensations for overdoing it. "No pain, no gain" is a phrase that was coined by Jane Fonda during her exercise guru years; however, Jane Fonda also openly admitted to having an eating disorder. So that concept was very Ed driven.

Besides physical symptoms, the psychological toll that compulsive exercise has is significant. As with food, obsessing about exercise pulls people away from their lives. It can create obsession as well as anxiety and depression if one is unable to engage in their compulsive behavior.

Daily exercise is important and necessary for overall health. However, if you are sick, it is more important to stay in bed and nurture yourself than to exercise. Exercising will make you sicker. This is about relearning how to treat your body with respect and give it what it needs. If you have the flu, a five-mile run certainly is not what you need. What you need is bed, hot tea, soup, sleep and a good book.

You don't need to be running like a banshee every single day. It's okay to alternate hard workouts with slower, less taxing workouts, such as aqua aerobics, or a leisurely walk through your neighborhood, a Hatha Yoga class, a Restorative Yoga class, or just playing at the playground with your kids or your friends' kids or kids you're babysitting for, or even going out dancing with your friends.

Rejecting your friends for exercise is the same as isolating with an eating disorder. You can become so incredibly obsessed with exercise, that your life is no longer your own. It's only about making sure that you get your fix. It's important to remain social and to get support from friends and people around you. It's very easy to isolate into an obsession. But all obsessions and disorders grow and thrive in isolation. As soon as support is given, they can be tamed.

It's okay to take a day off from exercise just because you don't feel like doing it. Like food, exercise needs to be something that keeps you healthy, not something that you obsess on and which makes you sick. All obsessions have the propensity to take over your life. Then, your life is no longer your own. You cease to make your own decisions; the obsession makes them for you. Ask yourself, "Am I making the decision to exercise, or is it the obsession that's driving it?"

If you suspect that you are addicted to exercise, and it's hurting you physically or emotionally, please tell someone. Many people don't understand that exercise can become harmful. So make sure that the person who you are talking to is safe and open to understanding what you might be going through. Talk to a therapist who specializes in treating eating disorders.

Figure out a plan that works for you. Try to take some days off and see what it's like for you, and what kind of emotions and fears and anxieties come up. Don't try to run away from the feelings or exercise them away; write about them and talk about them. You won't gain weight or get out of shape from skipping one day of exercise. That's just Ed talking to you. This is about integrating health and healthy ways of being in the world rather than being a slave to food, body image, and exercise and diets.

Step Thirty – Dealing with Desire and Wanting

It is common for people in their journey of recovery to feel like giving up. In fact, sometimes, it all hurts so badly that you might feel as if you've lost the motivation to recover. You might believe that you have to eat just to avoid the pain of not eating. You might feel as though food is the only thing you have to look forward to, and that it's easier to just give in to the binge. Why work so hard not to eat when, after all, food is consistent, food will never leave you, food is always there for you, you know that when you're feeling badly that you can just eat something and then you'll feel better.

Of course, the feeling that food gives you is temporary. That pint of Ben & Jerry's isn't going to fix your relationship issues or your money issues. True enough that you might feel some temporary relief, but it will rebound and you will feel worse. The relief is fleeting. But so are the feelings of giving up. Some days will be harder than others. Some days you will wake up feeling motivated and strong. Other days you will feel as though you just don't have it in you to recover. That's okay. These feelings will all pass. The need to binge will pass too, however strong it is. Just because you want to binge eat, doesn't mean you have to.

Hold that as a mantra: "Just because I want it doesn't mean I have to have it." I know it *feels* like you have to have it, but the truth is, you don't. You have to have air to breathe, you have to have food daily for nutrition, but you don't have to have a binge food.

So often, people believe that they need to satisfy their urges immediately. And why not? In this world, instant gratification is the norm. We demand that our urges be satisfied instantly. If they aren't, we become agitated. This is a fairly new phenomenon. People didn't always have 24-hour pizza delivery if they were craving a pizza at 3am. People didn't always have online porn that they could access at any time. We've become spoiled and unable to learn to sit with the feeling of wanting. The media sells directly to our compulsive sides because the feeling of wanting can be painful.

It is okay to want. But just because you want, just because you have an urge or an itch doesn't mean you have to satisfy it. You can *be in the wanting*. When the wanting is about food it is one of the easiest needs to satisfy. All you have to do is eat, and the wanting goes away. Fortunately, wanting food is the least painful want and is much easier to get past than a less tangible want to satisfy. For instance, it's heartbreaking to want to be with a certain person who rejects you. It's heartbreaking to want a child when you're unable to have one. It's heartbreaking to want your mother or father or husband or wife or child to be alive again. However, it's not heartbreaking to want a whole cheesecake or a gallon of ice cream. That want is fleeting, but it's a want that is simple to satisfy. Of course people often binge eat when they want something else that they can't have. For instance, sometimes, when people want something like money, a partner, a child, or love from a parent or spouse, they will eat. They have no control over how to get what they really want, but the want for food can be easily placated. After the want of food is satisfied, the other want still remains, and you still must learn to live with the pain of yearning after something that you have no control over.

When you find yourself in a place of wanting to binge eat, remind yourself: "Just because I want it doesn't mean I have to have it," and just sit with that for a little while. You might find that it wasn't actually food that you were craving.

The next time you find yourself wanting something that you don't have, notice what happens. Do you try to find something to eat? Do you wind up bingeing or compulsively eating something? If you find yourself grabbing for food, think about what you might actually be wanting. It is probably not food that is your true desire. Think about what you need and how you might be able to get support in that.

Sometimes your true desire is within your reach and there are ways to get what you want. Other times it is completely beyond your control but you can receive support from friends, family or a support group to get some nurturing for your pain. For instance, if you are feeling depressed because you wish you had more money, a way to help yourself with that would be to begin looking for a new job or looking for schools to go to. But if you are dealing with something that is beyond your control such as a diagnosis of a disease or disorder, or the loss of a loved one, it can be helpful to find other people who are going through similar issues for strength and support and to feel less alone. The pain of wanting is intensified by isolation. You certainly don't have to deal with pain alone. We were created as interdependent beings and we need each other. Allowing yourself to be vulnerable and asking for and receiving support is not weak, it's incredibly courageous.

Exercise One: Understanding Wants and Desires – *Journal Opportunity*

1. Something that I desperately want is:
2. When I think about this, I feel:
3. Wanting something that I can't have makes me feel:
4. Think about the last time you really wanted to binge, was there something else that you were really wanting?
5. If so, what was it?
6. What was going on for you when you thought about this thing that you wanted, what were you feeling?
7. What are some productive ways you might be supported in dealing with the pain of wanting?

Exercise Two: Feeling Gratitude for What You Do Have – *Journal Opportunity*

Getting rid of the uncomfortable pain of wanting is not necessarily an option. However, bringing in more pleasant feelings and gratitude for what you do have can make these feelings a bit more tolerable. One way to do that is with a gratitude list. A gratitude list is simply the old-fashioned notion of counting your blessings. One way to do this is to list out the things that you are grateful for in your life and then think of ways to bring more of this in. Here is an example of a gratitude list:

1. I am grateful for my awesome cat.
2. I am grateful for my apartment.
3. Even though I got laid off this year, I am grateful for the free time I have.
4. I am grateful for my best friend.
5. I am grateful for my intelligence.
6. I am grateful for my amazing roommate who is a great listener.
7. Even though she sometimes annoys me, I am grateful for my mom, who loves me too much sometimes.
8. I am grateful for the fact that I have a body that is healthy.
9. I am grateful for the color of my hair.
10. I am grateful for my ability to create art.

Now, how can you bring more of these things into your world?

1. I can pet my cat more and not take her for granted.
2. I can put beautiful things like flowers and handmade art up around my apartment and spend more time enjoying it.
3. I can take advantage of the free time I have now and do things like go to museums or do volunteer work.

4. I can spend more time with my best friend, and allow myself to enjoy her company.
5. I can read more and nurture my intelligence.
6. I can express my appreciation to my roommate for her amazing listening skills.
7. I can try to practice having more patience for my mom.
8. I can exercise, eat well and thank my body for supporting me.
9. I can stop complaining about my looks, and experiment with new and fun hairstyles.
10. I can take advantage of this talent and spend more time creating.

Name ten things that you're grateful for:

How can you bring more of this into your life?

I've often thought that getting outside of ourselves can be an amazing way to find some gratitude. One way of doing this is with volunteer work. Eating disorders can be so isolating, and just getting out and helping can create a space between you and the binge. It's also a great way to find some gratitude for the things that you do have.

Step Thirty-One – What if I Relapse?

A relapse is when, after cutting out a compulsive behavior, you engage in that behavior. So a binge relapse would be if you went several days or weeks or months or even years without a binge and then you binged. Relapses happen. Don't panic.

Progress is not linear. What's important after a relapse is how quickly you pull yourself out without fully falling into the disorder again. Rather than letting it take over you, you take over it. Relapses can be opportunities to learn more about yourself.

If you relapse, try to sit with it and examine it to figure out how it happened and what you could have done differently. When you relapse, sit and answer the following questions:

Exercise One: Understanding the Relapse – *Journal Opportunity*

1. This relapse occurred on:
2. Something that had been going on around that time was:
3. Something that I'd been thinking a lot about on that day was:
4. I was feeling this way on that day:
5. Aside from bingeing, what else could I have done to help me find some peace on that day, even to find peace around the anxiety of bingeing?
6. In the future, what warning signs will I have that a relapse is imminent?
7. What kind of plans and precautions can I take when those triggering times arise?

Relapses happen. The worse thing you can do when you relapse is to punish yourself for it. If you do, you will get stuck in it. Forgive yourself and move forward. For instance, don't continue bingeing and don't try to compensate by skipping meals or over-exercising to negate the binge. It will stick you back in the cycle of your Binge Eating Disorder again. Allow yourself to accept that relapses are a normal part of recovery. Get support for it and utilize the tools that you've gained up until now. It's okay. It happens to many people as they recover.

When you have a relapse, self-compassion is key. Understand that there might be something challenging going on in your life, which is why you binged in the first place. The irony is that when you binge eat, you are sending a signal to yourself that you need love and compassion, not anger and punishment. Yet, when people binge, they tend to berate themselves rather than give themselves the compassion and soothing that they need. Then begins a horrible cycle of bingeing, self-punishing and self-hatred and then bingeing again to diffuse the self-abuse.

You can learn from your setbacks. A binge doesn't happen when you begin eating a binge food. It actually starts several hours before. There is the point when you decide that you are going to binge that day. For some, there is a point when you decide several days in advance to binge. You plan it out for a certain event, post event, or just a day that you know you'll be alone. For many people, it's not that well thought out. Something happens early in the day and six hours later, they're knee deep in ice cream, seemingly winding up there without even realizing it. When you find yourself in this spot, it's time to do a *behavioral chain analysis*. In a behavioral chain analysis, we are looking at a sequence of events that led you to the behavior. If any link on the chain was different, how could the outcome have been different?

Though a binge can feel sudden and out of control, it has its roots in many hours or even many days before. For instance, you might wake up with a headache and feeling crabby, rather than eating breakfast you just grab some ibuprofen and a cup of coffee, you get to work late, your boss asks you to redo something that you know you'd done perfectly before. Your stomach is grumbling, you walk over to the vending machine and grab some chips. An hour later, you feel hungry again and go back to the machine and get another small bag of chips and this time a small bag of cookies. When lunchtime comes, rather than your usual soup and salad or sandwich, you grab a slice of pizza. That night, you come home from work and binge on ice cream. If you look at this day, there are several links in the chain that led to the binge. When you analyze it, you might be able to figure out who, what, where and how this happened, take responsibility for and think of new links that you could have added to the chain in order to have an outcome that was different. For instance, when you woke up in the morning you did not feel good. Rather than nurture yourself by either calling in to work and sleeping in a bit or eating a proper breakfast with your coffee and ibuprofen, you neglected your needs. When you got to work, you were still not feeling 100% and were vulnerable to your boss's criticism. Rather than chat with your boss about his or her criticisms – or even just taking some space from the office, or giving yourself positive self-talk – you found yourself too hungry and frustrated to make a healthy decision, so you grabbed chips and got to work. After working for a while, you found that you were still hungry and frustrated and grabbed some more junk food out of the vending machine. If at this point you'd allowed yourself a break and ate something healthy, you might have regained some sense of being in control or in power. But you were powerless against your boss's anger, powerless against your headache and powerless against the vending machine. By lunchtime, you already felt as though you'd failed that day and decided to just eat some pizza, promising yourself that you'd make better choices at dinner. When you got home that night you were grumpy, tired and just ready to soothe yourself and shake the day off. Although you did not actually binge during the day, you didn't make healthy choices for yourself and because you did not make healthy choices, you felt powerless, you felt like the day was a bust, you went into all or nothing thinking and decided that you'd make up for it by restricting the next day. At any point that day, you could have made a different decision. Even though you did not necessarily have the healthiest day with food, you still could have made the decision that night to go to a 12-step meeting or called a friend to talk out the day, or you could have decided to do something good for yourself, and taken a nice walk and prepared a healthy dinner that night. You could have made the decision at lunch not to have pizza, but to have a big salad and some protein in order to begin feeling healthier again. At any point you could have chosen a healthier 'link'. Unfortunately, unhealthy links attract unhealthy links, so it is up to you to notice and break that cycle. In this case, the binge did not start with the ice cream; it began hours before when you woke up with a headache. You might even take it a step further: why did you wake up with a headache? Did you drink too much wine the night before? Did you not get enough sleep? Were you dehydrated? What could you have done differently?

Exercise Two: Step-by-Step Behavioral Chain Analysis – *Journal Opportunity*

1. Describe the binge. Where did it happen? What time did it happen? What did you binge on? Was anyone else around? How much did you eat?
2. What were you feeling while you were bingeing?
3. How intense was the binge compared to other binges that you've had? Was it more intense, less intense? How did it compare?
4. Was there a particular event that you can point to that triggered the binge?
5. What happened just before the binge?
6. What happened an hour before the binge?
7. What happened earlier that day?

8. How were you feeling that day?

9. Did you try anything to prevent the binge?

10. What if any physical triggers were you feeling? (For example: did you eat a trigger food, or did you smell or pass a trigger food, were you very hungry, were you in any physical pain? Had you been restricting?)

11. Can you pinpoint when the binge sequence began?

12. What was going on for you emotionally the moment the sequence began? What were you doing, thinking, feeling, imagining at that time?

13. Was there anything that happened the day before that led into this day?

14. How was the day before or the last day that you did not binge different from this day?

15. What kind of *vulnerability factors* were involved with the binge, what made you more vulnerable to each link in the chain that led up to the binge? If you are unsure, the following four questions can help you answer that.

16. Were there physical factors such as pain or illness, hunger, fullness, lack of sleep, fatigue, or an injury; were there drugs or alcohol involved?

17. Was there some kind of external trigger such as a stressful event, stressful news, an argument or confrontation with someone?

18. Were you reacting to something that you learned, either positive or negative?

19. Did you have some kind of challenging emotion like anger, jealousy, sadness, fear or loneliness?

20. Were there previous behaviors that you acted out which triggered, stressed and built on this chain? For example, snacking on a food that you did not want to eat during a time when you were not hungry.

21. How did that link lead to the next link, which led to the next link, which eventually became the binge?

22. Link by link, describe how the chain of events led up to the binge.
23. Looking back at each link, what thoughts, feelings or beliefs did you have during and after each behavior?
24. Thinking about this objectively, as if you were directing someone other than yourself, what different links could you have injected into the sequence that could have created a more positive outcome?
25. Was there a solution at the end of any one of these links? Was bingeing a solution?
26. Did bingeing help at all? If so, how?
27. How could you have avoided bingeing?
28. Understanding what you know now about what you did, how could you prevent this in the future?

Step Thirty-Two – Understanding How Your Family Dynamics Have Influenced Your Binge Eating

Eating disorders aren't created in a vacuum. Your eating patterns were probably not established out of thin air. You did not choose to have an eating disorder because of an idea that came from nowhere. There are some obvious correlations like when parents criticize weight, as well as some not so obvious reasons.

Elaine, a 37-year-old patient of mine, had been battling with the starve/restriction cycle since she was in fourth grade. Her father, an avid athlete and health food nut, was perplexed when Elaine began to gain weight as a little girl. While she was certainly not fat, she was more developed than girls her age. She began to go through puberty early, got her period at age nine and developed very large breasts. Around that age, on a road trip with her dad, they stopped along the side of the road for lunch and Elaine ordered a sandwich with French fries and a cookie. Her dad looked from her to the food, with what she remembers as a disgusted look on his face, "Keep eating like that and you won't fit in the car... you're not such a little girl anymore." She felt horrible about herself. Not only was she suffering with the discomfort of an early puberty, but her father was rejecting her because of it.

"I felt disgusting," Elaine told me. "I had my period, I had breasts, I looked like a woman but I felt like a little girl. I felt like my father was rejecting me. I thought that he was telling me that I wasn't welcome in his car or in his life if I got fat, so I stopped eating." Elaine didn't eat her fries or her cookie and barely just picked at her sandwich. "Good girl," her father told her, "you'll be looking slim and trim in no time." To make matters worse, he had just remarried a woman with a daughter Elaine's age. She was a little pixie of a thing and as Elaine watched her father bonding with her new stepsister, she began to equate being worthy of love as being little. This began a cycle of severe restriction and extreme binges for Elaine.

"I used to go the whole day eating nothing but mustard out of a jar. As I got thinner and my parents gave me praise, I started to believe that I was only loveable when I was small." Of course this kind of eating wasn't sustainable for any length of time and Elaine would eventually steal food from the kitchen and hide in the closet while she binged on snack cakes. As she became an adult, these patterns remained. She would jump on the next new diet fad and shrink down 20–30 pounds and eventually start to binge and put it all back on. When she got into therapy and began addressing the feelings associated with how she grew up and her beliefs about being thin, she began to realize that she was loveable the way she was and didn't have to diet to gain love and respect. As she began to allow herself to eat, she found that she suffered less from the rebound binge and eventually not at all. Some cases are more extreme than that. For instance, when parents constantly pick on their kids' weight, put them on diets and restrict them from eating certain foods. I've heard of several cases where one child was put on a diet while the rest of the family, including the other kids, were allowed to eat whatever they wanted. Of course that never worked and these children mostly grew up to be overweight adults with sneak eating and binge eating issues.

While it's somewhat obvious that having an overly critical parent or a parent who was very focused on their child's weight would breed a child with an eating disorder, what about parents who were nothing but loving and supportive? What about families that never said a word about your weight or commented on what you did or how you acted or dressed?

What we have to remember about children is that they learn by watching. So, if you had a parent who was loving, kind and supportive to you, yet uncomfortable with his or her own looks, and was self-deprecating and constantly dieting, it would be challenging for you to have a strong self-esteem. This is because you didn't have a positive model for a healthy self-esteem.

Brianna was a 26-year-old former model. She came from a solid family, had an Ivy League education, earned a lot of money, had a kind and loving husband, but she secretly was bulimic. Each night after her husband was asleep, she snuck out of bed, found her binge foods that she kept stocked in a high cabinet that no one ever looked in, sat in the bathroom with boxes of cookies, bags of chocolates, candy and chips, binged on all of it, then would quickly purge it all. She would then clean herself off, brush her teeth, comb her hair, and slip back into bed with her husband and fall into a deep sleep. It was so separate and so compartmentalized from who she perceived herself to be and the person she projected out onto the world that she barely even noticed that she had a problem.

Brianna always described her family of origin as ideal. She gushed about their ski trips to Aspen, their annual Christmas party, their giant house, she extolled the relationship that she had with her parents and her sisters. She talked about how loving and supportive her family was. As our therapy went on and I prodded more, she began to discuss her mother's anxiety disorder and the cadre of meds that she was on. She told me that her mother would pick at herself constantly, never believing that she was good enough. She told me about her aunt's bipolar disorder and her suicide. When I asked how her family talked about feelings, and how they processed through the feelings of grief, loss and pain, she told me that they never discussed feelings at all.

So, even though Brianna didn't have an abusive or a critical family, things were swept under the rug, not discussed. Therefore, any discomfort that she had in life was repressed – literally stuffed down with food, and then expelled – purged. She had found a way with food to imitate the family's way of dealing with problems. Ignore. Her problems were in a little box not to be discussed or acknowledged, which is what made her bulimia so challenging to treat. It was incredibly challenging for her; but as she began to open up about what she was dealing with, the pain that she felt, she found that she was able to let go of her eating disorder. In fact, when she finally opened up to one of her sisters, her sister revealed that she suffered from Binge Eating Disorder and was in her own therapy to deal with it. Although the two were incredibly close and only two years apart, they didn't even know that one another were in treatment for eating disorders.

Exercise: How Has Your Family Contributed to Your Eating Disorder? – *Journal Opportunity*

Answer the following questions:

1. The following people commented on my body or eating habits:
2. What kinds of things did they say?
3. What kinds of beliefs did this lead you to have about your body?
4. What kinds of beliefs did this lead you to have about your own sense of worth?
5. When you think about this now, what do you feel?
6. How did your family discuss feelings?
7. What did you learn from this?
8. Is there a different way that you wish your family could have dealt with feelings?
9. If you could change something now about the way you acknowledge and discuss feelings, how would you do that?
10. When do you first remember having body image issues?
11. Did you tell anyone about it? How did they react?
12. When do you first remember dieting?

13. When do you first remember bingeing?
14. Was there anyone in your family who engaged in any kind of eating disordered behavior, for example: bingeing, obsessive dieting, food obsession, bulimia, compulsive behaviors around food, food hoarding, food restricting, anorexia, compulsive exercise, body image issues? If so, who?
15. What was that like for you? What did you think about it? How did it affect you when you were younger?
16. What did you learn from watching this behavior and how has it shaped your current beliefs?
17. If you could change your core beliefs and behavior, what would you change them to?

Beginning to understand how different family members all played a role in helping you to develop into the person that you have become is essential to healing. It helps you to remember that some thoughts you have just don't belong to you. That is not to say that you should be blaming your family for your eating disorder; these things are multigenerational and are passed down from family member to family member, and continue to grow and evolve as people integrate them into their lives. You can choose to heal generations of disordered eating and self-esteem issues and stop the cycle now through your own recovery.

Step Thirty-Three – Understanding Binge Eating in Your Relationship

Some couples are drinking buddies. They spend a lot of time going to bars or drinking at home together and alcohol becomes the third 'person' in their relationship. Often these couples aren't exactly sure what they'd do together if alcohol were not available. Clearly this can become problematic because of the inherent risks involved with frequent drinking. But what about when couples are eating buddies?

There are some relationships that revolve around food and eating. The couples plan elaborate vacations together where food and restaurants are at the center of their itineraries, they cook big elaborate meals together and they eat out together all the time. This can certainly be a lovely and meaningful common interest. However, there are couples where the obsession with food permeates every part of the relationship. They buy binge foods and sit home alone binge eating together. They diet together, vowing to stay away from certain foods, and then, as diets most often do, they fail together and begin bingeing again. The eating disorder becomes *triangulated* into their relationship. In family therapy, triangulation occurs when there is some kind of unspoken, unacknowledged conflict or unhappiness between two people. They then use a third person to mitigate that conflict. In this case, the Binge Eating Disorder has a personality. It is the third person in the relationship, thus forming a triangle.

When food is triangulated into a relationship, the couple will find that most of their conversations revolve around food – what they're eating, when they're going to eat, what they're going to eat. They might also have a great deal of conversations that revolve around their bodies and how to 'fix' them. They always have this common goal of losing weight, but rarely meet it.

The idea of grasping something that seems intangible bonds

them together. There is also the safety of having someone else who has the same challenges as you do, such as being a larger person in a world that celebrates being small or being unable to talk about uncomfortable feelings so turning to food to tune these feelings out.

Couples who triangulate food into their relationship will find that most of their social activities with each other revolve around food and food-related events. They will also find that if there is something going on in the relationship, some kind of conflict or something that one of them or both of them are unhappy about, that they will avoid the subject and try to get closer by isolating as a couple and eating together.

If one half of the couple begins to recover in a relationship like this, it can often be challenging for the other half, who might then feel threatened as they lose their partner in crime. It can also bring forth all the conflict that has been stuffed and avoided with food. There is also fear of losing the partner as they recover. Sometimes, partners find that without eating and food, they don't have much in common with each other, so each partner becomes invested in keeping one another in their disorder.

Is it possible that food might be triangulated into your relationship?

Are you and your partner obsessed with food?

Do you often do events together that revolve around food?

Do you binge and then vow to go on diets together then binge again? Is this a cycle?

Are you afraid that without eating, the two of you wouldn't have much in common?

Are there things in your relationship that go unspoken about?

Does one of you become threatened if the other begins a healthy lifestyle regimen?

Does one of you unconsciously try to sabotage the other when they begin a healthy lifestyle regimen, for example: bringing them binge foods or taking them to a restaurant where the food can be a binge trigger?

If this sounds familiar, some steps that you can take to detriangulate your relationship are:

- Talk about your feelings more with each other. When you each get home from work, set a timer and take 30–60 minutes without food, music, television, iPhones or computers present to discuss your days with one another.
- Begin to notice what role food plays in your relationship; for instance, if it's a Friday night and you've already eaten dinner and had dessert, but one of you decides that getting a pint of ice cream would be a good idea, discuss what it is that you're avoiding. Are you disinterested in being alone together without food? Are you afraid of what you would talk about or afraid that you might not have anything to talk about?
- Try to integrate some non-food activities into your relationship, like going to museums or art openings, or taking walks or some kind of (non-cooking) class together.

Getting into couples counseling is a great way to learn more about each other and learn how to talk about feelings with each other.

Step Thirty-Four – Tell Your Story

In recovery, when you tell your story to someone close to you or to a group of people or support group, you can find some catharsis, big change and transition as sharing helps you to find support from others and compassion from yourself.

You can use the following prompts to write your story, or just write it on your own – *Journal Opportunity*

The first time I remember thinking about food or my body…
Meals in my family were like this…
Food in my family was like this…
Body image in my family was like this…
The first time I binged:
I used to binge when:
My bingeing then evolved into:
I used food to:
I decided to start in recovery because:
This is how it's been going:

Try not to worry about how your story will be received, just concentrate on being honest with yourself and understanding your truth. You can't control what other people will think or how they will judge you, but you can control how you hold yourself. And you can do everything that you need to do to hold yourself with integrity. You can be the kind of person that you like. You can be the kind of person that you respect and admire.

Life is too short to waste time trying to make people like you. If they don't, keep being the good person that you are, and move on. You are perfect, whole and complete just being you. And each day, each moment, you can evolve more and more deeply into that whole being.

Appendix A: Further Resources

Visit the website at: http://www.reclaimingyourselffrombinge eating.com for tools, worksheets, journal prompts, and guided meditations.

Visit my blog, Recover http://www.bingeeatingtherapy.com for articles and tips on recovering from Binge Eating Disorder.

Online Tips and Help

http://www.dbtselfhelp.com/
http://psychcentral.com/
http://www.dailystrength.org/

Online Communities and Treatment Finders

ANAD – National Association of Anorexia and Associated Disorders
http://www.anad.org

Something Fishy – Eating Disorder Recovery Website
http://www.something-fishy.org/

ED Referral – Eating Disorder Referral and Information Center
http://www.edreferral.com

NEDA – National Eating Disorders Association
http://www.nationaleatingdisorders.org/

Pale Reflections – Online Eating Disorder Support Community
http://www.pale-reflections.com/

Health at Any Size – Support for health and well-being no matter what size you are
http://www.haescommunity.org/

Body Image Health – Tools for promoting health instead of size
http://bodyimagehealth.org/

Overcoming Overeating – An educational and training organization working to end body hatred and dieting
http://overcomingovereating.com/

Size Acceptance Association – Size-friendly activist community
http://www.size-acceptance.org/

Gurze Books – Eating Disorder Resources for Recovery
http://www.bulimia.com/

12-Step Groups for Eating Issues

Eating Disorders Anonymous
http://www.eatingdisordersanonymous.org/

Overeaters Anonymous
http://www.overeatersanonymous.org/

Anorexia and Bulimia Anonymous
http://aba12steps.org/

Food Addicts Anonymous
http://www.foodaddictsanonymous.org/

Compulsive Eaters Anonymous
http://www.ceahow.org/

Appendix B: Quick Tips to Stop a Binge in Its Tracks

Of course there will be times when you are about to binge or you are in the middle of a binge and feel that you can't stop. That is the time to HALT!

HALT is borrowed from 12-step groups.

Take a pause and think, am I:

H – hungry?
A – angry?
L – lonely?
T – tired?

Stop and try to calm yourself down. There are several ways to do this:

1. Your jaw is the strongest muscle in your body and as such it holds the most tension. If you need to release some tension, put a pillow over your mouth and scream as loud as you can into it. It's a great way to release stress.

2. Massage your jaw. You don't have to hold your mouth open, you don't have to hold it closed, let it fall into a neutral position and massage little circles into your jaw. This will help relax you.

3. The thymus tap: The theory is that tapping on your thymus helps to stimulate the immune system and elicits a calming response.

   How to do it: Make a fist and start tapping your fist on the middle of your chest, above your breastbone. The first tap is heavy, and the next two taps are a little softer. There is a pause between the first and second tap. So, the pattern is: tap, pause, tap, tap.

The tapping should be heavy enough to make a drumming sound in the chest. The vibration of the sternum caused by tapping helps to improve the thymus gland. Breathe naturally as you do the exercise, focusing on your breathing the entire time.

4. Take a deep breath into your belly. Breathe in slowly to the count of 5. Then, release to the count of 5. Do this 10 times. Your body should relax enough to give you some time to rationally decide whether or not this is what you really want to do.

5. EFT – Emotional Freedom Technique: This is tapping on acupressure points in order to let go of the urge to binge. Begin by assessing how badly, on a scale from 1–10, you want to binge.

    "My urge to binge is at a 10"

    Then, create an "even though" statement such as:

    > "Even though I want to eat all the cookies in the bag, I deeply completely accept myself."
    >
    > "Even though I have the urge to keep eating even though I'm full, I deeply completely accept myself."
    >
    > "Even though I (fill in what you feel), I deeply and completely accept myself."

    As you say this affirmation out loud, begin tapping certain points on your body. Tap lightly, enough that you feel it, but not so much that you hurt yourself.

    *   Tap the side of your hand and as you do, say your "even though" statement three times.

    Then, as you tap the pressure points, repeat the middle part of your even though statement. For instance: "want to binge on cookies, want to binge on cookies" as you continue to tap.

    *   Tap the outsides next to your eyes – near your temples
    *   Tap under your eyes

- Tap under your nose
- Tap under your mouth
- Tap under your collarbone
- Tap under your armpit next to your breast
- Tap the top of your head
- Tap the side of your hand again
- Tap inside your wrist
- Tap the top of your hand between your pinky and ring finger

Assess from a scale of 1–10 how badly you want to binge after you finish this cycle. Repeat this until you find some relief. For more information on the Emotional Freedom Technique, see emofree.com.

6. Postpone a binge with protein and a kitchen timer. When you are about to start eating, ask yourself, "Am I hungry?" If you are, let yourself eat a protein-dense food. If you're not, tell yourself that you are absolutely allowed to go and binge, but you are going to wait 20 minutes before you do anything. Set a timer for 20 minutes. Just sit and breathe for those 20 minutes or go for a walk. Tell yourself that you can come back when the buzzer rings if you still need to.

7. Find some distractions: This is the most popular post on my blog – 101 things that you can do instead of bingeing. Many of them don't require deep introspection or recovery activities. They're just straight up good healthy ways to distract yourself when you want to binge. Sometimes you might just be able to distract yourself right out of a binge.

   1) Call a friend, your sponsor, a support person, anyone who you can talk to who will either get your mind off of food, or someone to talk to about whatever it is that you might be feeling.

   2) Go for a walk.

3) Drink a cup of tea.
4) Take a relaxing bath with nice bath salts or essential oils.
5) Give yourself a manicure/pedicure – you can't binge with wet nails.
6) Volunteer at the SPCA to walk dogs or pet cats.
7) Go to a movie if the food there is not a trigger.
8) Watch a funny movie at home.
9) Take a shower, give yourself a hot oil treatment, shave your legs, tweeze your brows – self-care time.
10) Get organized: sort out your bills, create a budget – organize your home, your closet, your life! Often getting organized can help you feel more in control and enable you to thwart a binge, which can often feel very out of control.
11) Draw, paint or color.
12) Knit or do needlepoint.
13) Take a nap.
14) Get out of your house and into your car, go to the beach, the lake, the park... somewhere pretty and relaxing.
15) Clean out your closet, donate your old clothes or sell them on eBay.
16) Go window shopping.
17) Read a good book.
18) Clean!
19) Put on music and dance it out.
20) Go out dancing.
21) Call your friends over and have a dance party.
22) Go to the gym.
23) Stretch, go to a yoga class, do a yoga DVD or an exercise or yoga class on on-demand cable.
24) Meditate.
25) Write in your journal.

26) Move! Do jumping jacks, run in place, anything to move a little energy and release some tension.

27) Scream into a pillow.

28) Pray.

29) Go to a support meeting in person, online or on the phone.

30) Go to an online support forum with other people dealing with eating issues.

31) Read a (non-triggering) magazine.

32) Write a blog about your recovery journey.

33) Twitter!

34) Read personal journey blogs about others recovering from binge eating.

35) Sing!

36) Get your hair done or do your own hair. Experiment with different styles, curling iron, flat iron, curlers etc.

37) Make cards for people, catch up on Thank You notes, send out notes to relatives you haven't spoken to or seen in a long time.

38) Go out and take photos.

39) Scratch things off your 'to do' list.

40) Play video games.

41) Play scrabble online.

42) Chat with friends on Facebook or update your Facebook profile.

43) Write and direct a short play with stuffed animals or Barbie dolls or action figures or your pets or sock puppets and videotape it to put on the Internet.

44) Download MP3s.

45) Give yourself a foot massage.

46) Smell lavender or lavender oil – it has soothing properties.

47) Pick flowers.

48) Garden – a bacteria called Mycobacterium, which occurs naturally in soil, has the same effect on your brain as anti-depressant medications, so gardening if you enjoy it can be great for mental health – not to mention the benefit of getting out into the fresh air!

49) Create a collage.

50) Go bowling/miniature golfing.

51) Scrapbook.

52) Write an angry letter to whomever you are holding anger at. You don't have to send it, just let it out. Afterwards, put it somewhere safe. You might let go of some emotions that you'd been stuffing and you might find that you no longer have the urge to binge.

53) Go through old pictures.

54) Cuddle with your boyfriend, girlfriend, husband, wife, daughter, son, cat, dog, teddy bear etc.

55) Do karaoke, you can either go out to do it, or do it at home.

56) Water your plants and talk to them – if you don't have any, go out and buy some plants!

57) Go through your closet and donate all clothes that are too big, too small, out of date or unworn. Keep the clothes that you feel good about yourself in.

58) Zone out in front of the TV, catch up on your shows – as long as television is not a binge trigger.

59) Play music! If you play an instrument, whip it out and start playing. If not, teach yourself to play one. Beat on some bongos, ping a triangle, strum a guitar, whatever is convenient to you. If nothing, make an instrument out of household objects and play it. Being crafty is always helpful.

60) Tell the binge that you are stronger than it is. You are stronger than the urge to binge. Just because you want to, doesn't mean you have to.

61) Brush and floss your teeth.

62) Catch up on your e-mails.

63) Learn a new language.

64) Make a rubber band ball. Try to break the world record!

65) Write a letter to your future self, your recovered self, about what you're going through right now.

66) Write some notes with positive messages and post them around your home or get out of the house and put them up in dressing rooms, public restroom mirrors, restaurants, as does the organization Operation Beautiful!

67) Make a list of why you rock. Think about what's great about you. Can't think of those things? Call someone who loves you and ask them to tell you.

68) Spin around in circles like a Whirling Dervish. *Whirling Dervish (wurl-ing_dur-vish) n. 1. A mystical dancer who stands between the material and cosmic worlds. His dance is part of a sacred ceremony in which the dervish rotates in a precise rhythm. He represents the earth revolving on its axis while orbiting the sun. The purpose of the ritual whirling is for the dervish to empty himself of all distracting thoughts, placing him in trance; released from his body he conquers dizziness.

69) Light candles and incense and relax.

70) Explore your neighborhood or town.

71) Call a friend or relative who has been unhappy lately and needing some support. Sometimes giving support can be incredibly heartening and also supports the supporter.

72) Use crayons to color hard! This can release tension.

73) Build a terrarium.

74) Search through your couch and house for change! Put everything you can in a jar and put it aside to start a

fund for yourself as a motivator in your recovery.
Every time you reach a milestone (i.e. no bingeing or
restricting for one week) you can buy yourself
something fun, like a new pair of shoes, or some
jewelry or a new CD, or whatever you like within
reason.

75) Write a long, heart-wrenching letter and stick it in a
bottle and send it off.

76) Roll on your back. This is a spinal massage that helps
you to feel relaxed and rejuvenated.

77) Drink a glass of water.

78) Play solitaire.

79) Read or write positive affirmations.

80) Write out your intentions or personal goals for
yourself for the week. Write out both long-term and
short-term goals – things that you are striving for
and ways to help you get there.

81) Throw a temper tantrum! Go into your bedroom, lie
on your stomach in your bed and scream into your
pillow while you kick your legs and punch your
hands into the bed. Ever see kids do this? They
expend all that energy and it moves right through
them. As adults, we can't really do this and lots of
anger and pain winds up feeling stuck in the body.
We often try to stuff that down with food and, for
some, get rid of it by purging.

82) Plan a party or get together or weekend trip with
your friends.

83) Go bowling, play pool, play golf or miniature golf,
play basketball, hit tennis balls, go to a batting cage.

84) Beat up your pillow.

85) Make jewelry out of household items or beads or
coins.

86) Smell aromatherapy oils.

87) Paint old furniture.

88) Make stuffed animals or throw pillows out of old clothing.

89) Give yourself a facial treatment.

90) Look through old pictures.

91) Pretend that you are a tourist in your old city or town. Look up things to do that tourists would do and do them!

92) Teach yourself to juggle.

93) Go to the museum or the zoo. If it's not the right time, go to an online or virtual museum and learn all about art.

94) You can also take that old clothing, especially those items that are significant to your eating disorder days, and cut it up into squares and make a recovery quilt.

95) Write index cards with positive messages for yourself to look at when you're down.

96) Do a home makeover! Rearrange your furniture, get rid of things that you no longer want – sell them on eBay! Put up some curtains; just make things pretty for yourself.

97) Do online crossword puzzles, Sudoku or Boggle.

98) Enter sweepstakes.

99) Do volunteer work.

100) Write a novel, short story or poetry.

101) Fight procrastination by crossing things off your 'to do' list.

8. Find a mantra, and repeat it over and over. Some that I like:

- Just because I *want* to, doesn't mean I *have* to – the want will pass.
- I am stronger than the urge to binge.
- I am perfect, whole and complete just the way I am.

- I will feel worse later if I binge now, the satisfaction is so temporary.
- It's hard now, and I'm hurting, but I will feel better later.
- Every time I work through whatever is bothering me and avoid binge eating I become stronger, and the disease becomes weaker; I'm trying to get stronger.

Appendix C: PMS and Binge Eating

Many women notice that they are more likely to binge in the days before their periods. As your brain attempts to balance your hormones, you become deficient in serotonin. However, there are a few things that you can do to help balance your hormones.

Supplement with magnesium, Vitamin E, a B complex, Omega 3s and Omega 6s and Evening Primrose Oil. Take low dosage daily throughout the month. Even a potent vitamin mineral formula for women should be good.

Because there are so many hormones in meat and dairy products, if you can, switch to organic meat and dairy if it's viable for you.

Utilize an Edgar Cayce remedy by placing a castor oil pack over your liver during your time of the month. This is done by soaking a flannel cloth with castor oil and applying it to the lower right side of your abdomen. Cover the cloth with plastic wrap, and then apply a heating pad over this pack. You can just let yourself relax, maybe watch a fun movie or read a book while it's there. It should be very relaxing to you and supposedly will help to detoxify your liver and balance hormones.

Relaxation is key, because your body is working very hard during your time of the month and you will attempt to take care of yourself through food. Clearly, it's not the best medicine. Remind yourself that you are having PMS and that it's time to be gentle with yourself.

Appendix D: Supplements and Medication

Before starting a supplement regimen, check with your physician.

B Vitamins – help regulate serotonin levels to elevate mood and decrease binge episodes.

Chromium – 200 mcg per day – when needed for sugar cravings. Helps insulin to get into your cells to regulate glucose, so that your hormones stop sending messages to your brain that you need more sugar.

Manganese – 10 mg per day helps the transport and metabolism of glucose. It stabilizes blood sugar to reduce sugar cravings.

Magnesium – 500 mg per day – calms the body and the brain while stabilizing glucose levels which can wildly fluctuate when a person is binge eating. When magnesium levels are stable, cravings decrease.

Zinc – 15 mg – per day – helps to regulate appetite.

5-HTP – 200 mg per day in the evening – or whenever you have the urge to binge. The precursor to serotonin will suppress your appetite and relax you to take the anxiety away from the binge.

L-Glutamine – 500 mg when needed no more than 3 times per day. When you are having a strong sugar craving, take 500 mg of L-Glutamine or open a capsule and put the powder on your tongue. L-Glutamine is an amino acid that is converted into food for the brain.

Medication

At this point, there is no medication that has been approved expressly for the purpose of curing binge eating. However, there are some medications that have been prescribed off-label to treat Binge Eating Disorder:

Topamax – This anti-seizure medication is used to treat epilepsy.[12] According to a small 2002 study, 30 women were given Topamax and 31 a placebo. As compared to the placebo, Topamax was associated with a significantly greater rate of reduction in binge frequency, binge day frequency, body mass index, weight.[13] In a 2007 study using 400 subjects, half given placebo, half given Topamax, it was proven that the Topamax group both reduced obesity and decreased binge episode behaviors.

Wellbutrin – an SSRI (Selective Serotonin Reuptake Inhibitor), is an anti-depressant that is also used to help people quit smoking.[14] In three double-blind studies, it has been shown to reduce obesity. Anecdotally, many people report the side effect of weight loss when using Wellbutrin for other reasons.

Prozac – Prozac is approved by the USFDA to treat bulimia.

Appendix E: When You Feel Like Giving Up on Reading This Book

Wanting to give up on recovery is a totally natural and normal part of the recovery process. Though many people can start on a recovery process and go forward with it seamlessly, the majority of people struggle with recovery. Binge eating is a coping mechanism that has been constructed over a lifetime. Though it might have 'just' started a few years ago, it has its roots in childhood and how you learned to seek comfort, care and love. It takes time to unpack all this. And at times you need a break. You might want to just stop for a while. Perhaps giving yourself a time limit, like a week or a month, to take a break from recovery can be helpful. The most important thing is that you forgive yourself. Think about how many tries it takes people until they quit smoking. Or think about those addictive relationships where people break up and get back together over and over again until they finally end for good. Binge eating is just that, an addictive relationship with food. Sometimes it takes a few shots to give it up for good. If you can face and acknowledge what is happening though, you can understand why you want to give up. You might find that there is something underneath the feeling of wanting to give up your recovery that has nothing to do with the difficulty and challenge of it.

In your journal, ponder these questions when you feel as though you are ready to give up on this program:

1. I am ready to give up reading this book because I feel:
2. When I read this book, I feel:
3. When I do the exercises in this book, I feel:
4. I wish that I could recover by doing the following:
5. If I decide to stop trying to recover for a while, how might that benefit me?

6. If I decide to stop trying to recover for a while, how might that damage me?

7. What would it be like if I tried to persevere through my discomfort?

8. If I choose to stop working on this, how might I know when I will be ready to return?

9. How long will I choose my hiatus to be? A week? A month? Will it be permanent?

10. Is there a way that I can make this more palatable? Perhaps I'm doing too much of this? Perhaps I'm trying to jam it all in quickly? Can I do this slowly?

Even if you choose to stop working for a while, you cannot lose your recovery and unlearn what you have already learned. You cannot go backward, you can only go forward; and as you do progress, you will still have the tools with you that you need to recover, it is your choice as to whether you want to utilize them or not. You will still have a deeper understanding as to why you do what you do. This will always be helpful for you.

Appendix F: Tools

Alternative Action Log (Step Four)

Trigger: What Kind of Trigger was this, emotional, physical or situational?

_____

_____

_____

_____

_____

Describe What Happened:

_____

_____

_____

_____

Feelings: (What am I feeling about it?)

_____

_____

_____

_____

Short-Term Solution: (What do I want to do in the short-term to make me feel better?)

_____

_____

_____

_____

Long-Term Consequence: (How will that make me feel later, or tomorrow?)

_____

_____

_____

_____

_____

Alternative Behavior: (What else can I do to make myself feel better?)

_____

_____

_____

_____

_____

Feelings List

Pleasant Feelings:			Difficult/Unpleasant Feelings:		
Animated	Absorbed				
Open	Quiet	Anxious	Angry	Stupefied	A Sense of Loss
Happy	Accepting	Rebellious	Anxious	Forced	Tense
Alive	Festive	Devoted	Scared	Offensive	Boiling
Good	Spirited	Inquisitive	Depressed	Detestable	Fuming
Under-standing	Certain	Inspired	Lonely	Disillusioned	Indignant
Great	Kind	Unique	Confused	Hesitant	Indifferent
Playful	Ecstatic	Attracted	Helpless	Bitter	Indignant
Calm	Thrilled	Nosy	Irritated	Repugnant	Indifferent
Confident	Relaxed	Determined	Lousy	Unbelieving	Afraid
Gay	Satisfied	Dynamic	Upset	Despair	Hurt
Courageous	Wonderful	Passionate	Incapable	Aggressive	Sad
Peaceful	Serene	Snoopy	Enraged	Despicable	Insensitive
Reliable	Glad	Excited	Disappointed	Skeptical	Fearful
Joyous	Free and Easy	Tenacious	Doubtful	Frustrated	Crushed
Energetic	Laid Back	Admiration	Alone	Resentful	Tearful
At Ease	Cheerful	Engrossed	Hostile	Disgusting	Dull
Easy	Bright	Enthusiastic	Discouraged	Distrustful	Terrified
Lucky	Sunny	Hardy	Uncertain	Distressed	Tormented
Liberated	Blessed	Warm	Paralyzed	Inflamed	Sorrowful
Comfortable	Merry	Curious	Insulting	Abominable	Nonchalant
Amazed	Reassured	Bold	Ashamed	Misgiving	Suspicious
Fortunate	Elated	Secure	Indecisive	Woeful	Deprived
Optimistic	Jubilant	Touched	Fatigued	Provoked	Pained
Pleased	Love	Brave	Sore	Terrible	Neutral
Free	Interested	Sympathetic	Perplexed	Lost	Pained
Delighted	Positive	Empathic	Useless	Pathetic	Grief
Provocative	Strong	Brave and Daring	Annoyed	Incensed	Reserved

Encouraged	Loving	Loved	Diminished	In Despair	Alarmed
Sympathetic	Loving	Optimistic	Embarrassed	Unsure	Tortured
Overjoyed	Concerned	Comforted	Inferior	Tragic	Anguish
Impulsive	Eager	Validated	Upset	Infuriated	Weary
Clever	Impulsive	Drawn Toward	Guilty	Sulky	Panic
Interested	Considerate	Confident	Hesitant	Uneasy	Dejected
Gleeful	Affected	Hopeful	Vulnerable	In a Stew	Desolate
Free	Keen	Intent	Hateful	Cross	Bored
Surprised	Free	Certain	Dissatisfied	Bad	Nervous
Satisfied	Affectionate	Content	Shy	Pessimistic	Rejected
Thankful			Dominated	Desperate	
Receptive			Threatened	Preoccupied	
Fascinated			Appalled	Injured	
			Cowardly	Pessimistic	
			Humiliated	Cold	
			Quaking	Worried	
			Wronged	Offended	
			Menaced	Unhappy	
			Alienated	Disinterested	
			Wary	Frightened	
			Empty	Afflicted	
			Lifeless		
			Timid		
			Aching		
			Grieved		
			Shaky		
			Victimized		
			Mournful		
			Restless		
			Heartbroken		
			Dismayed		
			Doubtful		
			Agonized		

Food & Mood Log (Step Five)

HOW DO YOU FEEL PHYSICALLY BEFORE EATING?

_____

_____

_____

HOW DO YOU FEEL EMOTIONALLY BEFORE EATING?

_____

_____

_____

DESCRIBE YOUR LEVEL OF HUNGER BEFORE EATING – USE H/S SCALE:

_____

_____

_____

DESCRIBE WHAT YOU ATE INCLUDING SERVING SIZE:

_____

_____

_____

HOW DO YOU FEEL PHYSICALLY AFTER EATING?

_____

_____

_____

HOW DO YOU FEEL EMOTIONALLY AFTER EATING?

_____

_____

_____

DESCRIBE YOUR LEVEL OF HUNGER AFTER EATING:

_____

_____

_____

CHECK IN ONE HOUR LATER, HOW DO YOU FEEL NOW?

_____

_____

_____

Meal Planner (Step Eight)

Meal: Time: Place: Planned Food:

Hunger & Satiety Scale (Step Nine)

0   Starvation mode. Void of feelings. No energy, tired, empty.

1   Ravenous. Feeling uncomfortably hungry. Dizzy, grumpy.

2   Very Hungry, unable to focus on work or conversation.

3   Hungry. Stomach is beginning to growl; you are beginning to lose focus.

4   Getting Hungry. First thoughts of food begin.

5   Neutral. Not hungry, not full. Not obsessing about food. Nurtured, productive, able to focus. If you are eating, you can still eat more.

6   Satisfied. You've eaten enough to be content. You are not uncomfortable, yet you do not need more.

7   Slightly Full. A bit more than satisfied. You might feel like you had a bit too much.

8   Very Full. You begin to feel bloated as though you've had too much.

9   Uncomfortably Full. You just want to go to sleep. You might feel depressed or regretful.

10 Completely Stuffed. You feel like you might throw up. You are in pain, you can't focus, and you don't know how you got here.

0, 1, 2 & 8, 9, 10 – Danger Zone

3, 4, 5 – Go ahead and eat

6, 7 – Slow down, you can stop eating now

Automatic Thought Log (Step Nineteen)

1. What are you feeling? How strong are these feelings on a scale from 1–10?_____

_____

_____

_____

_____

_____

2. What are the thoughts that are triggering these feelings?_____

_____

_____

_____

_____

3. For each of these statements, what is absolutely true?_____

_____

_____

_____

_____

4. How do you know that's true?_____

_____

_____

_____

_____

5. Are there any thoughts here that might not be true?_____

_____

_____

_____

_____

_____

6. How do you know that these thoughts might not be true?____

_____

_____

_____

_____

_____

7. What is a more balanced truth here?_____

_____

_____

_____

_____

_____

8. What kind of cognitive distortion is this?_____

_____

_____

_____

_____

_____

9. How are you feeling now? How strong are these feelings on a scale from 1–10?_____

_____

_____

_____

_____

Critic Worksheet (Step Twenty-One)

Date & Time:_____

Event or Trigger (what happened):_____

_____

_____

_____

_____

What My Critic Said:_____

_____

_____

_____

_____

How that Made Me Feel:_____

_____

_____

_____

_____

How I Reacted or Behaved in Reaction to This: _____

_____

_____

_____

_____

Affirmation Creator (Step Twenty-Two)

The Goal You Want to Accomplish	The Affirmation to Help You Get There	The Eventual Affirmation

Affirmations

1. My body deserves love.
2. I am perfect, whole and complete just the way I am.
3. I feed my body healthy nourishing food and give it healthy nourishing exercise because it deserves to be taken care of.
4. I love and respect myself.
5. It's okay to love myself now as I continue to evolve.
6. My body is a temple. I want to treat it with love and respect.
7. My body is a gift.
8. Food doesn't have to be the enemy; it can be nurturing and healing.
9. Life is too short and too precious to waste time obsessing about my body. I am going to take care of it to the best of my ability and get out of my head and into the world.
10. I will not give in to the voices of my eating disorder that tell me I'm not okay. I will listen to the healthy voices that I do have, even if they are very quiet, so that I can understand that I am fine. I am fine.
11. Food doesn't make me feel better; it just temporarily stops me from feeling what I'm feeling.
12. I have everything inside of me that I need to take care of myself without using food.
13. A goal weight is an arbitrary number; how I feel is what's important.
14. I am worthy of love.
15. As long as I am good, kind and hold myself with integrity, it doesn't matter what other people think of me.
16. Other people are too busy thinking about themselves to care what my weight is.
17. When I compare myself to others, I destroy myself. I don't want to destroy myself so I'll just continue on my

journey, not worrying about other people's journeys.

18. I am blessed to be aging. The only alternative to aging is death.
19. It's okay for me to like myself. It's okay for me to love myself.
20. I have to be an advocate for me. I can't rely on anyone else to do that for me.
21. A 'perfect' body is one that works.
22. It's okay for me to trust the wisdom of my body.
23. Just because someone looks perfect on the outside, doesn't mean they have a perfect life. No one has a perfect life; we all struggle. That's just what being human is.
24. If I spend too much time trying to be and look like someone else, I cease to pay attention to myself, my virtues, my path and my journey.
25. When I look to others to dictate who I should be or how I should look, I reject who I am.
26. The last thing I should be doing is rejecting myself. Accepting myself as I am right now is the first step in changing, growing and evolving. When I reject myself, I cannot grow.
27. Self-respect is underrated.
28. I can only go forward, so although I can learn from it, I refuse to dwell on the past.
29. ALL images in magazines are airbrushed, photoshopped and distorted.
30. If people actively judge or insult me, it's because they feel badly about themselves. No one who feels good about themselves has the need to put someone down to elevate themselves – they have better things to do with their time.
31. I have no need to put someone down to elevate myself.
32. I can be a good person if I choose to be.
33. It's my life, I can choose the way I want to live it.
34. When I smile, I actually make other people happy.

35. Balance is the most important.
36. If I binge today, I can still love and accept myself; I don't have to beat, berate and starve myself right afterwards, and I still have the very next moment to jump right back into recovery.
37. Recovery is an ongoing process that is not linear in fashion. If I slip up, I'll take the opportunity as a learning experience and get right back to my recovery goals/program.
38. Progress is not linear. It's normal for me to go forward and then backward, and then forward again.
39. I enjoy feeling good. It's okay for me to feel good.
40. Having an eating disorder is not my identity.
41. Being skinny or fat is not my identity. I am identified by who I am on the inside, a loving, wonderful person.
42. I choose health and healing over diets and punishing myself.
43. My opinion of myself is the only one I truly know and it's the only one that counts. I can choose my opinion of myself.
44. When I am in my head too much, I can return to my breath, just breathe and be okay. There is only this moment.
45. It's okay to let others love me, why wouldn't they?
46. I am good stuff.
47. I am compassionate and warm. My presence is delightful to people.
48. My very existence makes the world a better place.
49. It's okay to pay someone to rub my feet every once in a while.
50. If I am hungry, I am supposed to let myself eat. Food is what keeps me alive.
51. Getting older makes me smarter.
52. It's okay not to be the best all the time.

53. My well-being is the most important thing to me. I am responsible for taking care of me. We are each responsible for ourselves.

54. No one has the power to make me feel bad about myself without my permission.

55. My feet are cute. Even if they're ugly.

56. I eat for energy and nourishment.

57. Chocolate is not the enemy. It's not my friend either. It's just chocolate: it has no power over me.

58. I can be conscious in my choices.

59. I am stronger than the urge to binge.

60. I am healthier than the urge to purge.

61. Restricting my food doesn't make me a better person; being kind to myself and to others makes me a better person.

62. Being skinny doesn't make me good. Being fat doesn't make me bad.

63. I can be healthy at any size.

64. Life doesn't start 10 pounds from now; it's already started. I can make the choice to include myself in it.

65. Food, drugs and alcohol are not the solution. They might seem like it at times, but using these things can make more problems. I have what I need inside of me as the solution.

66. There is a guide inside of me who is wise and will always be there to help me on my journey.

67. Sometimes sitting around and doing nothing is just what the doctor ordered. It's okay to let myself relax.

68. I am a human being, not a human doing. It's okay to *just be* sometimes. I don't always have to be doing.

69. My brain is my sexiest body part.

70. Looks last about five minutes – or until someone opens their mouth.

71. My life is what I make of it. I have all the power here.

72. My body is a vessel for my awesomeness.
73. My body can do awesome things.
74. If I am healthy, I am so very blessed.
75. I won't let magazines or the media tell me what I should look like. I look exactly the way I'm supposed to. I know because this is the way God made me!
76. What is *supposedly* pleasing to the eye is not always what is pleasing to the touch. Cuddly is good!
77. I can trust my intuition. It's here to guide me.
78. Just because I am taking care of myself and being an advocate for myself doesn't mean I'm selfish.
79. Not everyone has to like me. I just have to like me.
80. It's not about working on myself, it's about being okay with who I already am.
81. My needs are just as important as anyone else's.
82. Body, if you can love me for who I am, I promise to love you for who you are – no one is responsible for changing anyone else.
83. I will make peace with my body; it doesn't do anything but keep me alive and all I do is insult it and hurt it. I'm sorry body, you've tried to be good to me and care for me; it's time for me to try to be good back.
84. Thighs, thank you for carrying me.
85. Belly, thank you for holding in all my organs and helping me digest.
86. Skin, thank you for shielding and protecting me.
87. Other people don't dictate my choices for me; I know what's best for myself.
88. I feed my body life-affirming foods so that I can be healthy and vital.
89. Taking care of myself feels good.
90. I can eat a variety of foods for health and wellness without bingeing.
91. There is more to life than losing weight. I'm ready to

experience it.

92. If I let go of my obsession with food and my body weight, there is a whole world waiting for me to explore.

93. The numbers on the scale are irrelevant to who I am as a human.

94. Food is not good or bad. It has no moral significance. I can choose to be good or bad and it has nothing to do with the amount of calories or carbohydrates I eat.

95. I am still beautiful when I'm having a bad hair day.

96. My nose gives me the ability to breathe. Breath gives me the ability to be an amazingly grounded, solid person.

97. Being grounded and whole is what makes me beautiful. If I don't feel grounded and whole, I can get there just by being still, breathing, listening to my intuition, and doing what I can to be kind to myself and others.

98. I am not bad and I don't deserve to be punished, not by myself and not by others.

99. I deserve to be treated with love and respect and so do you. I choose to do and say kind things for and about myself, and for and about others.

100. Even if I don't see how pretty I am, there is someone who does. I am loved and admired. REALLY!

101. I promise myself today to live more from intention and less from habit.

102. "Beauty?... To me it is a word without sense because I do not know where its meaning comes from nor where it leads to." ~ Pablo Picasso

Recommendations for Further Reading

Mindfulness and Self-Acceptance:

McKay, M; Wood, J; Brantley, J (2007) *Dialectical Behavior Therapy Skills Workbook: Practical DBT Exercises for Learning Mindfulness, Interpersonal Effectiveness, Emotion Regulation, & Distress.* New Harbinger Publications

Brach, Tara (2004) *Radical Acceptance: Embracing Your Life With the Heart of a Buddha.* Bantam

Williams, M; Teasdale, J; Segal, Z; Kabat-Zinn, J (2007) *The Mindful Way Through Depression.* Guilford Press

Whole Food and Healthy Eating:

Planck, N (2007) *Real Food: What to Eat and Why.* Bloomsbury

Fallon, S (1999) *Nourishing Traditions: The Cookbook that Challenges Politically Correct Nutrition and the Diet Dictocrats.* NewTrends Publishing

Pollan, M (2007) *The Omnivores Dilemma: A Natural History of Four Meals.* Penguin

Eating Disorders:

Wachter, A; Marcus, M (1999) *The Don't Diet, Live It! Workbook: Healing Food, Weight, and Body Issues.* Gurze Books

Schaefer, J; Rutledge, T (2003) *Life Without Ed: How One Woman Declared Independence from Her Eating Disorder and How You Can Too.* McGraw-Hill

References

Chapter Four

Wise Mind

Linehan, MM (1993) *Skills Training Manual for Treating Borderline Personality Disorder*. New York Guilford Press

Shame

Brown, B (1997) *I Thought It Was Just Me (but it isn't): Telling the Truth About Perfectionism, Inadequacy, and Power*. Gotham

Gestalt

Perls, F (1973) *The Gestalt Approach & Eye Witness to Therapy*. Science and Behavior Books

Flaws of the BMI

Bacon, L (2010) *Health at Every Size: The Surprising Truth About Your Weight*. BenBella Books

Step Two:

Hara Hachi Bu

Reynolds, G (2011) *Presentation Zen: Simple Ideas on Presentation Design and Delivery*. New Riders

Step Seven:

B Vitamins

Chambers Clark, C (2004) *The Holistic Nursing Approach to Chronic Disease*. Springer Publishing Company

Step Nineteen:

Cognitive Restructuring

McKay, M; Davis, M; Fanning, P (2011) *Thoughts and Feelings: Taking Control of Your Moods and Your Life*. New Harbinger Publications

Endnotes

1. Hudson, JI; Hiripi, E; Pope, Jr., HG; Kessler, RC (2007) "The Prevalence and Correlates of Eating Disorders in the National Comorbidity Survey Replication." *Biological Psychiatry* 61(3): 348–58. doi:10.1016/j.biopsych.2006.03.040

2. Clara M. Davis and the wisdom of letting children choose their own diets. *CMAJ: Canadian Medical Association Journal* 2006 Nov 7; 175(10):1199–1201

3. "Clinical Spectrum of Obesity and Mutations in the Melanocortin 4 Receptor Gene." I. Sadaf Farooqi, MD, PhD; Julia M Keogh, BSc; Giles SH Yeo, PhD; Emma J Lank, BSc; Tim Cheetham, MD; and Stephen O'Rahilly, MD. *N Engl J Med* 2003; 348:1085–1095 March 20, 2003

4. "The Regulation of Body Weight". Martin, Roy J; White, B Douglas; and Hulsey, Martin G. *American Scientist* Vol. 79, No. 6 (November–December 1991), pp. 528–541

5. "Evidence for sugar addiction: Behavioral and neurochemical effects of intermittent, excessive sugar intake." Avena, Nicole M; Rada, Pedro; Hoebel, Bartley G. *Neurosci Biobehav Rev.* 2008; 32(1): 20–39. E-pub 2007 May 18

6. "Food addiction and obesity: evidence from bench to bedside." Liu, Y; von Deneen, KM; Kobeissy, FH; Gold, MS. *J Psychoactive Drugs.* 2010 Jun; 42(2): 133–45

7. "Reduced serotonin transporter binding in binge eating women." Kuikka, Jyrki T; Tammela, Liisa; Karhunen, Leila; Rissanen, Aila; Bergström, Kim A; Naukkarinen, Hannu;

Vanninen, Esko; Karhu, Jari; Lappalainen, Raimo; Repo-Tiihonen, Eila; Tiihonen, Jari; Uusitupa, Matti. *Psychopharmacology* 2001 May Vol. 155(3): 310–314

8. "The effect of food deprivation on brain and gastrointestinal tissue levels of tryptophan, serotonin, 5-hydroxyindoleacetic acid, and melatonin." Bubenik, George A; Ball, Ronald O; Pang, Shiu-Fun. *Journal of Pineal Research* 1992 Jan; 12(1): 7–16

9. "Obesity, binge eating and psychopathology: Are they related?" Christy F. Telch, PhD, Staff Psychologist, W. Stewart Agras, MD, Professor of Psychiatry. *International Journal of Eating Disorders* Volume 15, Issue 1, pp. 53–61, January 1994

10. "Kleptomania, compulsive buying, and binge-eating disorder." McElroy, Susan L; Keck, Paul E; Phillips, Katherine A. *Journal of Clinical Psychiatry*, 1995; 56 Suppl 4:14–26

11. "Differences in serotonin transporter binding affinity in patients with major depressive disorder and night eating syndrome." Lundgren, JD; Amsterdam, J; Newberg, A; Allison, KC; Wintering, N; Stunkard, AJ. *Eat Weight Disord.* 2009 Mar; 14(1):45–50

12. The *American Journal of Psychiatry (Am J Psychiatry)* Vol. 160 Issue 2, pp. 255–61 (Feb 2003) ISSN: 0002-953X [Print] United States

13. *Biological Psychiatry (Biol Psychiatry)* 2007 May 1; 61(9): 1039–48. ISSN: 0006-3223 [Print] United States

14. Li, Z; Maglione, M; Tu, W; Mojica, W; Arterburn, D; Shugarman, LR; Hilton, L; Suttorp, M; Solomon, V; Shekelle, PG; Morton, SC. (2005). "Meta-analysis: pharmacologic treatment of obesity." *Ann Intern Med* 142(7): 532–46. PMID 15809465

About the Author

Leora Fulvio, MFT, is a licensed Psychotherapist and Hypnotherapist practicing in San Francisco. She has been treating women with food and body image issues since 1999. She studied Creative Writing at Bard College and received her Masters of Counseling Psychology at the California Institute of Integral Studies. She is passionate about helping women heal from the tyranny of eating disorders and self-reproach. When she is not working with clients or writing, she enjoys relaxing with her husband and sons.

AYNI
BOOKS

"Ayni" is a Quechua word meaning "reciprocity" – sharing, giving and receiving – whatever you give out comes back to you. To be in Ayni is to be in balance, harmony and right relationship with oneself and nature, of which we are all an intrinsic part. Complementary and Alternative approaches to health and well-being essentially follow a holistic model, within which one is given support and encouragement to move towards a state of balance, true health and wholeness, ultimately leading to the awareness of one's unique place in the Universal jigsaw of life – Ayni, in fact.